Extreme Rapid Weight Loss Hypnosis

Powerful Mini Habits that Stop Emotional Eating, Trigger Calorie Blast, Create Perfect Portion Control Effortlessly, and Boost Your Self Esteem

Robert Williams

Table of Contents

Introduction

Rapid weight loss hypnosis is a very advanced level hypnosis recording that is designed to help you lose weight super fast, but the most important thing is that it doesn't involve starvation. This system has been extremely effective for me and others in the past. It is also designed to help you lose weight in a healthy non-harmful way so that you can maintain your weight-loss lifestyle in the long term.

I personally got to a very unhealthy weight, which I managed to lose using this system. There is no way I could have done it without this system because it is a very powerful one. I'm now more than the healthy weight I wanted to be and I'm now wearing the clothes I always wanted to wear. My life has completely changed thanks to this method.

The principle behind this program is very, very simple, but it does require a little bit of discipline because it is based on how your body naturally works. When you eat food your body needs to digest it, but when you first start to feel hungry again, you've probably only just started to digest the first meal. So, if you don't eat again, your body doesn't have enough time to digest, so that's why you feel hungry and you feel a lack of energy. So by not eating, you're giving your body extra time to digest and gives you more energy.

And when you haven't eaten for a while your metabolism will increase and you will lose weight.

The trick to this is to not eat too much before you sleep—for example, if you do it at the wrong time (i.e, too much before sleeping), you will feel hungry before you go to sleep and it will delay your sleep for a long time and you will probably end up feeling tired the next day.

Another crucial thing is to drink lots of water.

This is why I strongly recommend you have a very healthy daily routine and daily exercise program, too. If you can integrate the two, you will maximize your weight loss results.

The extreme rapid weight loss hypnosis itself is designed to stimulate a desire to sleep and relax so that your mind is clear to absorb the weight loss messages. It is a very advanced hypnosis recording for weight loss, designed to keep you eating less and not eating before you go to sleep. This is actually very important because if you eat unnecessarily your body doesn't have enough time (sleep) to digest it properly, so in the long run, it can cause long-term health problems. This doesn't apply if you are very hungry and you eat without listening to this recording, but not too often.

What is Self-Hypnosis for?

It was Milton H. Erickson, founder of modern hypnotherapy, who gave an exhaustive illustration of the effects and purposes of hypnosis and self-hypnosis. The scholar stated that this practice aims to communicate with the subconscious of the subjects through the use of metaphors and stories full of symbolic meanings (Tyrrell, 2014).

If incorrectly applied, self-hypnosis can certainly not harm, but it may not be useful in attaining the desired results, with the risk of not feeling motivated to continue a constructive relationship with the unconscious. However, to do it as efficiently as possible, we need to be in a relaxed state of mind. So, accordingly, we start with relaxation to gather the attention inside, while suspending conscious control. Then we insert suggestions and affirmations to the unconscious mind. At the end of the time allocated for the process, a gradual awakening procedure facilitates the return to the state of permanent consciousness. When you are calm, your subconscious is 20-25% more programmable than when you are agitated. Also, it effectively relieves stress (you can repair a lot of information and stimuli you understand), aids regeneration, energizes, triggers positive physiological changes, improves concentration, helps you find solutions, and helps you make the right decisions. If the state of conscious trance is reached, then if the patient manages to let himself go by concentrating on the words of the hypnotist, progressively forgetting the external stimuli, then the physiological parameters undergo considerable variations. The confirmation comes from science, and in fact, it was found that during hypnosis, the left hemisphere, the rational one, decreases its activity in favor of the more creative hemisphere, the right one (Harris, n. d.).

You can do self-hypnosis in faster and more immediate ways, even during the various daily activities after you have experienced what state you need to reach during hypnosis.

A better understanding of communication with the unconscious mind highlights how indispensable our collaboration is to slip into the state outside the ordinary consciousness. In other words, we enter an altered state of consciousness because we want it, and every form of hypnosis, even if induced by someone else, is always self-hypnosis.

We wish to access the extraordinary power of unconscious creativity; for this, we understand that it is necessary to put aside for a while the control of the rational mind and let ourselves slip entirely into relaxation and into the magical world of the unconscious where everything is possible.

Immense benefits can be obtained from a relationship that becomes natural and habitual with one's own unconscious. Self-hypnosis favors the emergence of constructive responses from our being, can allow us to know ourselves better, helps us to be more aware of our potential, and abler to express them and use them to foster our success in every field of possible application.

How Do You Do Self-Hypnosis?

There are several self-hypnosis techniques out there; however, they are all based on one concept: focusing on a single idea, object, image, or word. This is the key that opens the door to trance. You can achieve focus in many ways, which is the reason why there are so many different techniques that can be applied. After a period of initial learning, those who have learned a method, and have continued to practice it, realize that they can skip certain steps. In this part, we will take a look at the essential self-hypnosis techniques.

The Betty Erickson Method

Here I'll summarize the most practical points of this method of Betty Erickson, wife of Milton Erickson, the most famous hypnotist of 1900.

Choose something you don't like about yourself. Turn it into an image, and then turn this image into a positive one. If you don't like your body shape, take a picture of your body, then turn it into an image of your beautiful self with a body you would like to have. Before inducing self-hypnosis, give yourself a time limit before hypnotizing yourself by mentally or better yet, saying aloud the following sentence, "I induce self-hypnosis for X minutes." Your mind will take time like a Swiss watch.

How Do You Practice?

Take three objects around you, preferably small and bright, like a door handle, a light spot on a painting, etc., and fix your attention on each one of them. Take three sounds from your environment, traffic, fridge noise, etc., and fix your attention on each one. Take three sensations you are feeling, the itchy nose, tingling in the leg, the feeling of air passing through the nose, etc. It's better to use unusual sensations, to which attention is not usually drawn, such as the sensation of the right foot inside the shoe. Don't fix your attention for too long, just enough to make you aware of what you are seeing, feeling, or trying. The mind is quick. Then, in the same way, switch to two objects, two sounds, two sensations. Always be calm, while switching to an object, a sound, a sensation. If you have done things correctly, you are in a trance, ready for the next step.

Now let your mind wander, as you did in class when the teacher spoke and you looked out of the window, and you were in another place, in another time, in another space, in a place where you would have liked to be, so completely forget about everything else. Now recall the initial image. Perhaps the mind wanders, from time to time it gets distracted, maybe it goes adrift, but it doesn't matter. As soon as you can, take the initial image, and start working on it. Do not make efforts to try to remind you of what it means or what it is. Your mind works according to mental associations, let it work at its best without unnecessarily disturbing it: it knows what it must do. Manipulate the image, play with it a little. See if it looks brighter, or if it is smaller, or it is more pleasant. If it is a moving image, send it back and forth in slow motion or speed it up. When the initial image always gets worse, replace it instantly with the second image.

Chapter 1:   Benefits of Hypnosis

Using Hypnosis to Encourage Healthy Lifestyle Changes

In addition to helping you encourage yourself to eat healthier while discouraging yourself from eating unhealthy foods, you can also use hypnosis to help encourage you to make healthy lifestyle changes. This can support you with everything from exercising more frequently to picking up more active hobbies that support your wellbeing in general.

You may also use this to help you eliminate hobbies or experiences from your life that may encourage unhealthy dietary habits in the first place. For example, if you tend to binge eat when you are stressed out, you might use hypnosis to help you navigate stress more effectively so that you are less likely to binge eat when you are feeling stressed out. If you tend to eat when you are feeling emotional or bored, you can use hypnosis to help you change those behaviors, too.

Hypnosis can be used to change virtually any area of your life that motivates you to eat unhealthily, or otherwise neglect self-care to the point where you are sabotaging yourself from healthy weight loss. It truly is an incredibly versatile practice that you can rely on that will help you with weight loss, as well as help you with creating a healthier lifestyle in general.

With hypnosis, there are countless ways that you can improve the quality of your life, making it an incredibly helpful practice for you to rely on.

The Benefits of Hypnotherapy for Weight Loss

It is hard to pinpoint the single best benefit that comes from using hypnosis as a way to engage in weight loss. Hypnosis is a natural, lasting, and deeply impactful weight loss habit that you can use to completely change the way you approach weight loss, and food in general, for the rest of your life.

With hypnosis, you are not ingesting anything that results in hypnosis working. Instead, you are simply listening to guided hypnosis meditations that help you transform the way your subconscious mind works. As you change the way your subconscious mind works, you will find yourself not even having cravings or unhealthy food urges in the first place. This means no more fighting against your desires, yo-yo dieting, "falling off the wagon," or experiencing any inner conflict around your eating patterns, or your weight loss exercises that are helping you lose the weight. Instead, you will begin to have an entirely new mindset and perspective around weight loss that leads to you having more success in losing weight and keeping it off for good.

In addition to hypnosis itself being effective, you can also combine hypnosis with any other weight loss strategy you are using. Changed dietary behaviors, exercise routines, any medications you may be taking with the advisement of your medical practitioner, and any other weight loss practices you may be engaging in can all safely be done with hypnosis. By including hypnosis in your existing weight loss routines, you can improve your effectiveness and rapidly increase the success you experience in your weight loss patterns.

Finally, hypnosis can be beneficial for many things beyond weight loss. One of the side effects that you will probably notice once you start using hypnosis to help change your weight loss experience is that you also experience a boost in your confidence, self-esteem, and general feelings of positivity. Many people who use hypnosis regularly find themselves feeling more positive and in better spirits in general. This means that not only will you lose weight, but you will also feel incredible and will have a happy and positive mood as well.

If you can afford to undergo a series of hypnotherapy sessions with a specialist, you may do so. This is ideal as you will work with a professional who can guide you through the treatment and will also provide you with valuable advice on nutrition and exercises.

Clinical Hypnotherapy

When first meeting with a therapist, they start by explaining to you the type of hypnotherapy he or she is using. Then you will discuss your personal goals so the therapist can better understand your motivations.

The formal session will start with your therapist, speaking in a gentle and soothing voice. This will help you relax and feel safe during the entire therapy.

Once your mind is more receptive, the therapist will start suggesting ways that can help you modify your exercise or eating habits as well as other ways to help you reach your weight loss goals.

Specific words or repetition of particular phrases can help you at this stage. The therapist may also help you in visualizing the body image you want, which is one effective technique in hypnotherapy.

To end the session, the therapist will bring you out from the hypnotic stage, and you will start to be more alert. Your personal goals will influence the duration of the hypnotherapy sessions as well as the number of total sessions that you may need. Most people begin to see results in as few as two to four sessions.

DIY Hypnotherapy

If you are not comfortable working with a professional hypnotherapist or you can't afford the sessions, you can choose to perform self-hypnosis. While this is not as effective as the sessions under a professional, you can still try it and see if it can help you with your weight loss goals.

Here are the steps if you wish to practice self-hypnosis:

1. Believe in the power of hypnotism. Remember, this alternative treatment requires the person to be open and willing. It will not work for you if your mind is already set against it.
2. Find a comfortable and quiet room to practice hypnotherapy. Ideally, you should find a place that is free from noise and where

no one can disturb you. Wear loose clothes and set relaxing music to help in setting up the mood.

3. Find a focal point. Choose an object in a room that you can focus on. Use your concentration on this object so you can start clearing your mind of all thoughts.

4. Breathe deeply. Start with five deep breaths, inhaling through your nose and exhaling through your mouth.

5. Close your eyes. Think about your eyelids becoming heavy and just let them close slowly.

6. Imagine that all stress and tension are coming out of your body. Let this feeling move down from your head, to your shoulders, to your chest, to your arms, to your stomach, to your legs, and finally to your feet.

7. Clear your mind. When you are relaxed, your account must be clear, and you can initiate the process of self-hypnotism.

8. Visualize a pendulum. In your mind, picture a moving swing. The movement of the pendulum is popular imagery used in hypnotism to encourage focus.

9. Start visualizing your ideal body image and size. This should help you instill in your subconscious the importance of a healthy diet and exercise.

10. Suggest to yourself to avoid unhealthy food and start exercising regularly. You can use a particular mantra such as "I will exercise at least three times a week. Unhealthy food will make me sick."

11. Wake up. Once you have achieved what you want during hypnosis, you must wake yourself. Start by counting back from one to 10 and wake up when you reach 10.

Remember, a healthy diet doesn't mean that you have to reduce your food intake significantly. Just cut your consumption of food that is not healthy for you. Never hypnotize yourself out of eating. Only suggest to yourself to eat less of the food that you know is just making you fat.

Chapter 2: Gastric Band with Hypnosis

Many different types of hypnosis benefit the human body in different ways. Some of these methods include hypnosis for weight loss and healthy living, which are different types of hypnosis for weight loss. Gastric band hypnotherapy is one of them and popularly known as a type of hypnotic state that is suggested to your subconscious, which involves fitting a gastric band around your stomach. This in return helps you lose weight, along with general hypnosis for weight loss sessions.

This type of hypnotherapy is often considered as the final type of hypnotherapy people try if they would like to reach their goals. The practice involves surgery known as gastric band surgery. During surgery, a gastric band gets fitted around the upper part of your stomach, with the purpose to limit the total amount of food you consume daily. This is a more extreme type of hypnotherapy for weight loss, which has proven to help people lose weight. Since it is surgical, you cannot carry out this method yourself. It also includes potential risks, which is why it must be treated with respect and only carried out by a certified medical practitioner.

You can, however, implement gastric band hypnotherapy yourself. It is a technique most commonly used by hypnotherapists with the purpose to trick the subconscious into believing that a gastric band has been fitted when in reality it hasn't. Since hypnotherapy is focused on putting your

23

conscious mind silent, and implementing thoughts and beliefs in your subconscious mind, as a type of hypnotherapy, it is quite effective. Given that hypnotherapy offers us many benefits, as well as allows us to imagine and come to terms with what we are capable of doing, it acts as the perfect solution to reaching some of your goals that may seem out of reach.

Gastric band hypnotherapy involves the process of believing that you have experienced the physical surgery itself, ultimately making you believe that the size of your stomach itself has been reduced too.

The gastric band used in gastric band fitting surgery is an adjustable silicone structure, used as a device to lose weight. This gastric band is used during surgery and placed strategically around the top part of your stomach, leaving a small space above the device. The space left open above the gastric band restricts the total amount of food that is stored inside the stomach. This is done to implement proper portion control every day and prevents overeating. The fitted gastric band physically makes it difficult for one to consume large amounts of food, which can set you in the habit of implementing proper portion control daily. This will essentially cause you to feel fuller after eating less, which in return encourages weight loss.

Most people choose to have the surgery after they've tried other methods to lose weight, including yo-yo dieting, diet supplements, or over-the-counter drugs, all with the hope to lose weight. Gastric band surgery acts as a final resort for those who desperately want to lose weight and have been struggling for a long time.

Gastric band hypnotherapy serves as a very useful method as it can allow you to obtain a similar result as the gastric band fitting surgery itself. That's because you are literally visualizing getting the same procedure done and how you benefit from it. During gastric band hypnosis, you are visualizing yourself losing weight subconsciously, which translates into your conscious reality.

Hypnotherapists that specialize in gastric band hypnotherapy focus on finding the root of what prevents their clients from losing weight. Most of the time, they discover that emotional eating is one of the leading causes that contribute to people holding on to their weight. They also make a point of addressing experiences that remain in your subconscious mind but are yet to be addressed. These experiences often cause people to turn toward unmindful and emotional eating, which then develops into a pattern that feels impossible to kick.

Since stress is added to our lives every day, and people don't stop and take the time to process feelings or perhaps not even give it a thought, most turn to food for comfort. This also plays into emotional eating, which has extremely negative effects on the body long-term as it also contributes to one of the leading causes of obesity.

Given that obesity is an incredibly bad illness and more people get diagnosed with the condition every day, it is something that needs to be addressed. If gastric band hypnotherapy can prevent it or restructure our thinking patterns to not act on our emotions, but rather invite and process them, then it is a solution that everyone who needs to lose weight should try.

Once a hypnotherapist learns about why you're struggling to implement proper portion control, they will address it with the virtual gastric band treatment at a subconscious level. During this visualization session, you will have imagined that you have undergone the operation and had the gastric band placed around your upper stomach. This will lead you to think that you feel fuller quicker, serving as a safer option as opposed to the surgery.

How Gastric Band Hypnotherapy Works

Hypnotherapy for weight loss, particularly for portion control, is great because it allows you to focus on creating a healthier version of yourself safely.

When gastric band fitted surgery gets recommended to people, usually because diets, weight loss supplements, and workout routines don't seem to work for them, they may become skeptical about getting the surgery done.

Nobody wants to undergo unnecessary surgery, and you shouldn't have to, either. Just because you struggle to stick to a diet, workout routine, or lack motivation, does not mean that an extreme procedure like surgery, is the only option. In fact, thinking that it is the only option you have left, is crazy.

Some hypnotherapists suggest that diets don't work at all. Well, if you're motivated and find it easy to stick to a diet plan and workout routine, then you should be fine. However, if you're suffering from obesity or overweight and don't have the necessary drive and motivation needed, then you're likely to fail. When people find the courage and determination to recognize that they need to lose weight or actually push themselves to do it, but continuously fail, that's when they tend to give up.

Gastric band hypnotherapy uses relaxation techniques, which are designed to alter your way of thinking about the weight you need to lose, provides you a foundation to stand on and reach your goals, and also constantly reminds you of why you're indeed doing what you're doing. It is necessary to develop your way of thinking past where you're at in this current moment, and evolve far beyond your expectations.

Diets are also more focused on temporary lifestyle changes rather than permanent and sustainable ones, which is why it isn't considered realistic at all. Unless you change your mind, you will always remain in a rut that involves first losing, and then possibly gaining weight back repeatedly. Some may even throw in the towel completely.

Since your mind is incredibly powerful, it will allow you to accept any ideas or suggestions made during your gastric band hypnosis session. This can result in changing your behavior permanently as the ideas practiced during the session will translate into the reality of your conscious mind. By educating yourself on healthy habits, proper nutrition, and exercise, you also stand a better chance of reaching your weight loss goals sustainably.

The gastric band fitting procedure will require a consultation with your hypnotherapist where you will discuss what it is you would like to gain from hypnotherapy. After establishing your current health status, positive and negative habits, lifestyle, daily struggles, and goals, they will recommend the duration of hypnotherapy you will require to see results. During this time, you need to inform your hypnotherapist of your diet and physical activity history. They are likely to ask you questions about your current lifestyle and whether you changed it over the years. If you've lived a healthy lifestyle before, then they will try to find and address the reasons why you let go of yourself and your health. If you have always lived your current unhealthy and unbalanced lifestyle, they will trace it back through the years with the hope to discover the reasons behind it. During your initial session, your weight loss attempts, eating habits, and any health issues you may experience will be addressed. Your attitude toward food will also be acknowledged, as well as your relationship with it, with people, and your surroundings.

Now your therapist will have a better idea of the type of treatment you need. The procedure is designed to have you experience the gastric band surgery subconsciously, as though it has really taken place. You will be talked to in a deep, relaxed state, exactly the same as standard hypnosis. During this session, you will be aware of everything happening around you. Suggestions to help boost your self-esteem and confidence are often also incorporated into the session, which can also assist you in what you would like to achieve consciously.

You will be taken through the procedure step-by-step. Your hypnotherapist may also make theater noises to convince your subconscious even more. After your session, your hypnotherapist may give you self-hypnosis guides and techniques to help you practice a similar session for the results to become more effective. Sometimes, gastric band hypnotherapy only requires a few sessions, depending on what your needs are.

Gastric band hypnosis doesn't only involve having to go to physical hypnotherapy sessions, but it also requires you to implement some type of weight management program that specifically addresses your nutrition, addiction, and exercise habits. It addresses habits between your body and mind and helps you implement new constructive ones.

After gastric band hypnosis, you can expect to feel as though you have a much healthier relationship with food, as well as a more mindful approach in everything you do. During the visualization process of gastric band fitting surgery, you will come to believe that your stomach has shrunk, which will trick your brain to think that you need less food. This will also make you think that you don't need a lot of food, which will make you more acquainted with consuming healthier portion sizes.

Gastric band hypnotherapy is successful as it makes you think that you are full after eating the daily recommended amount of food for your body. It is also considered much healthier than overeating or binge eating. You will learn to recognize the sensation of hunger versus being full, which will help you articulate between the two and cultivate healthier eating habits.

Chapter 3:   How Hypnosis Works

Understanding Hypnosis

For over 200 years, individuals have been contemplating and contending about hypnosis, yet science still needs to explain how it really happens, completely. We see what an individual is doing under a trance, yet why the individual is doing it isn't obvious. Ultimately, this riddle is a little piece in a lot bigger riddle: how the human personality works. It is far-fetched that specialists within a reasonable timeframe will think of authoritative clarification of the brain. So it is safe to say that the phenomenon of hypnosis will further remain a mystery.

Be that as it may, specialists know the general aspects of hypnosis. As such, they have some examples of how it functions. It is a condition of stupor portrayed by serious suggestive, unwinding, and expanded dream. It is unlike sleep since the individual is alert at all times. On the other hand, wandering off into fantasy land, or the feeling of "losing yourself" in a book or film, is generally common. You are completely mindful. However, most of the environment around you is blocked out. Focus seriously on the current point.

In the day-to-day daze of ordinary life, an evoked universe seems to some extent genuine to you, as it connects completely with your feelings. Specific occasions can trigger genuine dread, misery, or satisfaction, and in case you're stunned by something (for instance, a beast hopping out of the shadows), you may even shake in your seat. That is why most analysts characterize every single daze as self-trance of sorts.

Milton Erickson, the twentieth century's driving master in sleep induction, contended that people are mesmerized every day. In any case, most specialists focus on the condition of daze brought about by purposeful unwinding and thinking workouts. This significant mesmerizing is frequently compared among alertness and rest to the casual mental state.

In a standard trance, as though they were the truth, you approach the trance specialist's recommendations or your considerations. On the chance that the trance inducer demonstrates your tongue has swollen up to twice its size, you will feel an inclination in your mouth, and you may experience issues talking. In case you're drinking a chocolate milkshake, the trance specialist demonstrates, you'll taste the milkshake and feel it cooling your mouth and throat. If you are frightened, the subliminal specialist shows, you may feel panicky or start perspiring. Yet, constantly, you know it's everything fanciful. As youngsters do, you "play imagining" on an extraordinary level.

Individuals feel uninhibited and agreeable in this specific mental state. This is most likely because they settle the worries and questions that normally hold their exercises under tight restraints. While watching a film, you may encounter a similar impression; as you get inundated in the plot, worries about your work, family, and so on blur away, until all you're considering is what's on the screen.

You're likewise amazingly suggestible in this state. That is, if the subliminal specialist advises you to accomplish something, you are probably going to embrace the idea completely. This is the thing that makes it so agreeable to demonstrate the stage subliminal specialist. Delicate grown-ups are typically held to stroll around the stage all of a sudden, clucking like chickens or singing as loud as possible. There is, by all accounts, the dread of humiliation flying out the window. Nonetheless, the suspicion that all is the well and good and ethical quality of the subject stays installed all through the experience. You can't get a subliminal specialist to do anything you would prefer not to do.

How Does Hypnosis Work?

A certified trance specialist or subliminal specialist prompts a condition of serious fixation or concentrated consideration during trance. This is a strategy guided by verbal signs and redundancy.

In numerous regards, the stupor like the state you enter may appear to be like rest, yet you are completely aware of what's going on.

Your advisor will make guided proposals to help you achieve your restorative goals while you are in this stupor-like state. Since you are in an increased center state, you might be increasingly open to recommendations or proposals that you may incur negligence or get over in your standard mental state.

Your advisor will wake you up at the end of the session from the stupor-like state, or you will leave. It's dubious the impact this extraordinary focus level and thought consideration have. During the daze-like state,

32

hypnotherapy may situate the seeds of unmistakable thoughts in your psyche, and rapidly those changes flourish and thrive.

Hypnotherapy can likewise make ready for more profound treatment and acknowledgment. In the event your brain is "jumbled" in your day-by-day mental expression, your psyche will most likely be unable to retain proposals and counsel.

What Happens to the Brain During a Hypnotic Session?

Harvard scientists examined 57 individuals' cerebrums during guided trance. They found that: two mind areas in charge of handling and controlling what's going on in your body during mesmerizing show higher movement.

Thus, during entrancing, the locale of your mind that is responsible for your activities and the area that is aware of those activities have all the earmarks of being separated.

Is Everything Only a Misleading Impact?

It is possible, yet in the brain's action, trance shows checked differentiations. This shows the mind reacts unmistakably to spellbinding, one that is more grounded than fake treatment.

Like spellbinding, recommendation drives the misleading impact. Guided discourses or any type of social treatment can strongly affect lead and feelings. Entrancing is one of those instruments of treatment.

Do Reactions or Dangers Exist?

Mesmerizing infrequently makes or displays risks to any reactions. It tends to be a safe elective treatment decision as long as the treatment is performed by a certified subliminal specialist or trance inducer.

A few people may encounter gentle to direct symptoms, including cerebral pain tiredness, unsteadiness situational uneasiness. However, an antagonistic practice is spellbindingly utilized for memory recovery. People who consequently use spellbinding are bound to encounter nervousness, misery, and opposite reactions. You may likewise have a more noteworthy possibility of making false recollections.

Chapter 4:   Hypnosis and Weight Loss

Part of being human means that you have feelings. At times, you may feel more emotional than other times. Some of these emotions can lead us to emotional eating. You find that all you want to do is keep eating even when you are not hungry. This is an unhealthy eating habit that can cost result in weight gain or at times, lead to some diseases. Meditation allows you to take charge of your emotions. Instead of regularly being emotional, it allows one to find some solutions for the challenges that they are facing. As you focus your mind on analyzing them, you can easily come up with a possible solution.

Helps You Avoid Overeating

You might have been hungry the whole day, and all that you are looking forward to is laying your hands on a sumptuous meal. You find that you have invested your mind into thinking a lot about the food you want to consume. When you do that, your appetite increases. Once you get a meal, you end up overeating since your mind has already registered that you were really hungry. Regardless of the amount of food you consume, you have the urge to keep taking more. In the process, you end up overeating and regretting late. At times, sweet food can make us overeat. It might be one of those good days where you are feeling energetic, and you get to cook a nice meal. You spend much of your time making the meal, and when it comes to eating it, you find yourself overeating since it is a delicious meal. Meditation allows you to know when you are full, and hence you get to

35

understand that there is no need to keep adding more food. You get to eat the portion that you need, and you can save the rest for another day. In this case, it allows you to have self-control as you consume your food.

You Find Other Ways to Reduce Stress

Stress eating is a major challenge among a variety of people. Life can get challenging, and you feel like you are under pressure. There are different challenges that we face. Some of them are beyond our control while others are manageable. You might have recently lost a loved one. The loss makes you feel stressed, and you may wonder why they had to go. An individual might be in a situation where they feel lonely, and this results in stress. On the other hand, you might have failed a test and you feel bad about the whole situation. You might probably be wondering if you will manage to graduate in the intended year or if you will have to stay longer at school. These are some of the situations that cause stress. When they occur, your solution might be eating. Anytime you feel sad or feel like crying; you end up looking for a meal to eat. In this process, you end up overeating, and the food consumed is not helpful to your body. Meditation allows you to come up with ways of handling such stressful situations and hence, one no longer needs to overeat.

It Allows You to Cope with Eating Disorders

Some individuals have chronic eating problems, such as bulimia and anorexia. Individuals with anorexia tend to deny themselves food. You find that they eat little portions of food in a day, which is lower than the amount of food their body needs. You find that some people struggling with weight gain tend to be anorexic. With weight gain, their self-esteem lowers, and they develop other complications. At times they may be uncomfortable around some individuals, and anytime they consume anything, all they want to do is throw up and release the food consumed. We also have some models struggling with anorexia. They want to be a certain shape, and hence they lower their food intake. They do not consume the required food portions, and it can have some harmful effects on their bodies. Bulimia refers to a condition whereby the individual consumes a lot of food, which is unnecessary. This is a challenge to petite individuals who want to add extra weight. You find that regardless of the amount of food that they consume, no big change occurs in their body. Meditation allows you to accept yourself as you are and hence, you do not need food to boost your self-esteem.

It Improves Focus

When your mind is in a calm state, your concentration level increases. You find that you become more focused on the task that you are undertaking, and you do it well. Eating requires some focus. For instance, while chewing, being focus can help you in the proper chewing of food. In this case, all the food particles are well broken down. This makes certain processes such as digestion easier. When this occurs, the food consumed is well utilized in the body. In this case, all the food becomes beneficial, and none is wasted. It also makes the process of ingestion easier. The challenge of having excessive and unutilized foods in the body is managed. As a result, the problems that result from poor eating are also well taken care of. Focus is essential in all aspects of life. It improves our performance

37

in the tasks that we are undertaking, and it ensures that we make the right choices. You might overlook the importance of focus when it comes to eating, but it plays a crucial role.

You Eat Only the Required Food Portions

In some moments, greed causes us to eat more food than we require. Greed can result from seeing a good well-prepared meal and automatically desiring to have it. You might have eaten, and you were full, but since you came across a meal that looks delicious, you have the sudden urge to consume it. In that case, you will be eating not because you are hungry, but due to greed. To avoid some of those incidences, you need to have some self-control. When you have consumed the needed portion of food, you have to train your body not to need more. Even if you eat the extra portion, it has no purpose to your body since the body does not use it. It instead disposes of waste since it does not add any value to it. At times your body will convert it into fat, and you end up gaining weight. On the other hand, some people misunderstand the concept of dieting and think that it means denying themselves food. You may find that an individual is skipping some meals just to lose weight. When you do this, you deny your body its needs, and it can result in further complications. To avoid this, ensure that you take the required amount of food.

It Allows You to Avoid Impulse Buying of Food

Impulse buying of food is similar to impulse shopping. In impulse shopping, you find that you are walking around a shop to buy a specific item, but you end up buying items that you had not budgeted for. For instance, you might be walking to a supermarket to buy some groceries, but you end up buying a pair of shoes. You had no intention of getting the shoes, which means it is an added item to your budget. On the other hand, you might find yourself not using the item you bought because you did not need it in the first place. Such random purchases also occur with food. As you are walking along the streets, you may come across a fast food joint, and you automatically decide to get some fries. You initially did not have any plans to get them, but since you came across them, immediately, a need arises. Meditation allows you to make the right choices. You get to analyze the situation and decide on the best thing to do. In most cases, you will decide to forego making the impulse purchase

Helps in Self-Awareness

We have been created to function differently. Each individual has their own unique characteristics that set them apart from the others and make them who they are. Your way of thinking and doing things might be different from that of another person. At times you will get in an interview, and they tell you to describe yourself. What are the responses you would have to give? Most people freeze when asked this question because we are not aware of who we are. We barely take time to understand ourselves, and hence we know little about who we are. Meditation allows us to connect with our inner being. When you take some me-time, you may decide to meditate about your life. This will involve asking yourself some important questions and your responses to the asked questions will tell a lot about the kind of person that you are. When it comes to acquiring healthy eating habits, self-awareness is necessary. You need to be well aware of the challenges that you will face while trying to adapt to some of those eating habits. This allows you to easily focus and manage to successfully utilize the good eating habits.

Helps You Follow Your Diet Plan

Following a diet plan can be quite a challenging task. The first days can be challenging, especially if you have never tried it before. You may decide to have only one meal that is out of the diet, and you end up having more than just one meal. Instead of the one meal that you had promised yourself, you extend it to a week, and before you know it, you are no longer following the diet plan. While dieting, you will need a lot of discipline that ensures you stay focused on your decisions. Despite the circumstances or the events around you, you always ensure that you stay focused on what you do. The biggest challenge with dieting is that you will always come across food. As you walk across different streets, you will come across food. You could also be sitting near an individual who is eating, and you feel tempted to get what they are eating. It takes a lot of discipline and self-control to ensure that you stick to your diet. Meditation allows you to acquire this kind of discipline and it ensures that you stay focused on your goals and plan.

Chapter 5:   Risks of Rapid Weight Loss Hypnosis

There are several risks associated with obesity. Heart disease, cholesterol, and diabetes are just some of the dangers of overweight. However, losing weight isn't the easiest thing to do. People with weight issues are continually losing their pounds and putting them on again. Is it any wonder that crash diets for rapid weight loss are becoming so popular? Rapid weight loss is something people's overweight are hoping for. But is there some fast weight loss program that could shave off the pounds and hold them off? What's more, losing weight is a super-fast idea? What are the health risks?

Yeah, these are some of the questions that should come to your mind when you look at commercials for fast weight loss programs. It could be tempting to look at a quick weight loss plan that means you're looking at a 20-pound slimmer reflection of yourself in a week, but don't give in to that temptation. The benefits of rapid weight loss may not be irreversible, and you may do irreparable harm to your metabolism. Thus, the positive effects cannot last long, but the detrimental effects can end up haunting you forever.

If you are already susceptible to kidney issues, trying to lose weight quickly might make them worse. You can end up with gall bladder stones or low blood pressure, as well as mineral imbalances in your body. None of this

42

will bode well for your wellbeing in the long run. Adding to this is the chance that you will regain all your lost weight within a few months of losing it. While some people profit from accelerated weight loss programs, the findings have not always favored the plan. Oprah Winfrey was a case in point a few years back when she woke us after losing weight to the oodles, but she put it all on again in a short time.

The quickest weight loss program appears to require you to starve yourself. This way is not the way to lose weight. Bear in mind that if you deprive yourself, you run the risk of binging yourself. So, you might end up eating a lot more than you've been dreaming about. The result: all the pounds you've lost will be back again. There is also a high risk that you will develop an eating disorder.

How do you plan to eradicate those pounds and hold them off? Eat right and exercise right. Many people prefer to go from overweight to slim to overweight again because they set unrealistic weight-loss expectations. The intention is to slow down but to keep going towards that objective. The quickest way to ensure that you do this is by adopting a healthy diet. Eat fats; eat carbohydrates; ingest those calories—just don't stuff yourself with them. Schedule yourself for a daily workout, drink a lot of water, and have a nice rest. Soon, you should be looking at a slimmer you minus the consequences of a rapid weight loss.

Being overweight is something that almost any person in the world is trying to stop. This way is incredibly right given the number of health hazards that one is exposed to while he or she is overweight and the issues with self-esteem that come with not being in shape. It is, therefore, not shocking that weight-loss diets and fat-loss exercises are standard in the world today. However, to shed extra fat, some people typically use techniques that help them lose weight fast, which is generally to the detriment of their bodies. The following are the hazards to which one is subjected as he or she attempts to lose weight quickly.

It is usually recommended that one should make sure that he or she does not lose more than 2 lbs a week. Any weight loss of more than 2 lbs. is generally considered risky as it typically exposes a person's body to significant health risks. This way is because rapid fat loss typically denies the body the time it requires to adapt to weight loss and therefore creates instability in the body's metabolic system, which can often have disastrous implications.

Losing weight with hypnosis is one of the fastest, quickest, and safest and most calming, and cheapest ways to lose weight permanently. I've been hypnotizing thousands of people for more than 17 years, and I haven't seen someone who tries to make this work fail for them when they try to do what they're supposed to do. There have been many independent studies on weight-loss communities in many different ways, from medications to special diets, but none has performed as well as hypnosis. If you understand hypnosis and know what to expect, you're going to be effective in losing all the weight you want, and you need to lose, even if you don't believe it's going to work, it's going to work anyway. Hypnosis is working if you want it to work. Anyone can be hypnotized if they want to. You'll lose weight if you're going to lose weight. The only thing that can save you from being hypnotized is you. I've got people telling me, "I don't think I can be hypnotized." They're usually my best customers. They're usually people who have some significant myths about hypnosis and may have tried it, but nothing magical happened, so they gave up. They just want it to work, but they just didn't know how to do it until they were better informed about hypnosis.

There are some basic facts about hypnosis that you need to know. When someone with experience hypnotizes you, you'll sit back and relax, close your eyes and listen to the hypnotherapist's voice to guide you. There's nothing you can do wrong; nothing can go wrong. There are no risks in this form of hypnosis. All hypnosis is self-hypnosis. You're still in charge of that. You're never going to do or say anything against your will, interests, values, or principles, regardless of what others think. It's like a mental test or a mind game. And you're not losing hold of your thoughts. You're still in charge of that. You're not losing your hearing or any of your senses. In reality, your senses become sharper, and you become more conscious, not less. You're still going to hear me whether you think you do it or not. You're doing all the work, and all the work is in your head. You don't have to say something or do something about it. The hypnotherapist uses their experience to guide you through your head, to send you guidance, but you don't have to follow them if you're not comfortable with any part of it. There's no sense in being hypnotized. You're not going to be hypnotized. The only thing you're going to experience is sort of comfortable to really comfortable. Others get just a little comfortable and listen to every word and remember it all, whereas others are so comfortable, they snorkel. Still, nobody can sleep until you're at home in bed for the night, and you're exhausted anyway when you put on your CD. Often it may feel like sleep, but it's not sleeping. All the work is in your head, so you have to take part and think about what the hypnotherapist suggests. It's just a guided meditation and incredibly strong.

With Hypnosis, you will be able to achieve your perfect weight and figure. You're going to lose all the weight you want and need to lose, without tension and emotional challenges with cravings, impulses, overfeeding, stuffing yourself as you do when you diet. It's not a diet, but you're not going to put your weight back on! You don't feel like you're starving, though you're looking for more nutritious, lower-calorie, healthy foods. You won't want the rich, fattening, unhealthy, high calories, candy, unhealthy food, and food that isn't good for you. You're not going to snack or eat between meals or late at night. You're going to eat what your body wants, and when you're satisfied, you're fully satisfied. You won't lose weight as easily as it might damage your health. You will concentrate on the perfect shape and scale and achieve the ideal size quickly and without discomfort and keep that size as long as you want. You're going to want to drink more water and be happy from one meal to the next. You're going to lose weight without trying! Your eating habits can change suddenly, instantly, or gradually over time. Some people will be hypnotized once, and their eating habits will change forever, and others need to be hypnotized.

Chapter 6:   Hypnotherapy for Weight Loss

Because it plunges into a second and modified state of consciousness, hypnosis is a particularly interesting approach in the case of overweight. The idea? Allow you to access your subconscious to reprogram it.

Despite drastic lifestyle changes and a good dose of motivation, it is sometimes difficult to get rid of certain well-established eating habits. By dint of repeated regimes that do not give lasting results, frustration sets in and we very often end up getting discouraged and giving up.

Hypnosis for losing weight is therapeutic hypnosis (hypnotherapy), called Ericksonian. It should not be confused with "spectacle" hypnosis during which the practitioner takes control of his subject. Focused on relaxation, hypnosis for weight loss is a very different approach. During the session, you remain conscious and perfectly in control of yourself. The hypnotherapist is there to guide you gently and help you better understand where the eating behaviors that cause your weight gain come from. By this serene journey to the heart of your subconscious, you deeply modify certain conditioning and bad eating habits.

Alternative medicine par excellence, hypnosis for losing weight is a powerful tool that will allow you to (re) take control and regain your ideal weight durably and without frustration.

47

Hypnosis to Help Overweight

From a scientific point of view, several studies have shown the effectiveness of hypnosis on several disorders:

- Peptic ulcer
- Tinnitus
- Spathic colitis
- Itching/eczema
- Chronic migraines
- Certain allergies
- Certain forms of bronchitis asthma
- Spasmophilia
- Phobias
- Sexual problems
- Addiction
- Anxiety attacks
- Insomnia

This gentle therapeutic approach has proven itself, both in terms of physical health and psycho-emotional balance. Often, eating behaviors that promote weight gain is a matter of stress and managing emotions. We even speak of "emotional pounds."

Moreover, when we are going through a particularly stressful period, two main trends emerge, loss of appetite or, conversely, the need to consume caloric foods, rich in sugars and fats.

Because it allows this altered state of consciousness and promotes letting go, hypnosis for losing weight gives real results and allows better management of overweight linked to stress. In particular, it helps to:

- Alleviate the anxiety that causes compulsive eating and snacking
- Get rid of food addictions
- Take over when temptation is present
- Hunt complexes and regain self-confidence
- Strengthen your mind and motivation

Lasting Weight Loss with Hypnosis

Of course, losing weight necessarily involves questioning one's eating habits. Since we have to go through this, it is legitimate to wonder how hypnosis for losing weight concretely triggers these changes in perception. During the session, the therapist immerses his patient in a very deep state of relaxation. His goal encourages him to access his subconscious mind and certain automatisms/conditioning which are the cause of his bad eating habits. Accompanied by the voice of the hypnotherapist, the patient deconstructs his relationship to food. This is, for example, to suggest to his subconscious that high-calorie foods are not the only ones that do him good.

This deep introspective work is the guarantee of lasting weight loss. Losing weight through hypnosis, therefore, meets the expectations of those who seek to lose weight permanently... without going through the frustration box!

Effectiveness of Hypnosis Session for Losing Weight

What to Expect

The idea of losing weight with hypnosis arouses your curiosity? Because we all have the spectacular spectacle hypnosis in mind, we very often associate this practice with a total loss of control.

Provided by a qualified hypnotherapist, a hypnosis session to lose weight lasts 1 hour and leaves you entirely free to move and think. First stage? An essential exchange that will allow your practitioner to identify your problem and personalize this hypnosis session to lose weight.

With relaxation techniques, your therapist guides you to a deep state of letting go. This hypnotic state, known as a second and modified state, will then allow you to gain gentle access to your unconscious and the conditioning responsible for your weight gain.

If the voice and the expertise of the practitioner accompany you throughout the session, it is you who walk in the heart of your subconscious and are the actor of these deep inner changes.

More and more people recognize the benefits of hypnosis to help people lose weight and maintain a healthy and stable weight over time. Beyond simple testimonials, there are scientific studies that prove the effectiveness of hypnotherapy. One of the first studies on this subject, conducted in 1986, showed that overweight women who used a hypnosis program lost significantly more weight (about 8 kg) than those who were simply told to be careful what they ate. Another study showed that women who used hypnosis to lose weight had slimmed down, improved their body mass index, changed their eating behaviors, and even developed a more positive body image.

In the accompaniment of weight loss, the hypnotherapist is a kind of coach, who will first of all help his patient to enter a state of deep relaxation. Once this state is acquired, the hypnotherapist will be able to access the patient's subconscious, which is more open to suggestions than the conscious part of the mind. The hypnotherapist seeks to break the bad eating habits of the patient by replacing the patterns of thought that lead to overeating with more positive and balanced attitudes in relation to food, through visualizations and suggestions.

Thus, hypnotherapy is an approach to weight loss that is based on a change in the relationship with food in the long term: it is to change the way of thinking of the patient, so that these thoughts are translated into healthier actions vis-à-vis its diet. Hypnotherapy is therefore not for those who are looking for "miracle" solutions: it is a process that is certainly effective but takes time. Changing a patient's attitude towards food requires a good knowledge of the particular problems of the food, and the development of suggestions that respond exactly to his problems. Thus, the first step in any hypnosis for weight loss is going to be a conversation between the therapist and his patient, so that the latter explains his history in terms of diets, what has helped or complicated his weight loss before, etc. Thus, any person thinking of hypnosis as a weight-loss technique must abandon the express attitude that accompanies many diets: it is a therapy aimed at a total change in lifestyle and behavior towards feed screw.

Thus, thanks to the power of suggestion, the hypnotherapist can replace negative thoughts and unhealthy behaviors by redirecting them towards actions better for the health of the individual: the hypnotherapist will in no case propose a diet, but helps to adopt a new way of life. Hypnosis helps people to deal with psychological problems that can explain bad lifestyle habits, such as hatred of sports, excessive greediness, binge eating, etc. It is used to identify the psychological concerns that trigger these bad habits, to correct them, and create more positive patterns. So, one of the key aspects of hypnotherapy's work in weight loss is going to be to convince the patient that he can lose weight and that these past failures do not affect the possibility of present success. A big problem with people trying to lose weight repeatedly is that they think their bad habits are "stronger" than they are: the hypnotherapist helps chase away those negative thoughts.

In connection with this, behavioral and cognitive therapy, which is done with the accompaniment of a mental health professional, can be an excellent complement to hypnotherapy. This type of psychotherapy allows the patient to talk about feelings and thoughts that he has with food, which allows him to be fully aware of the thought patterns and problems at the source of his unhealthy relationship with his diet. Subsequently, it will be easier for him to change their habits. Indeed, being aware of the problem is the first step towards more appropriate habits.

Another advantage of hypnotherapy for weight loss is that it can also help individuals to better manage their stress. Thus, faced with difficult everyday situations, the individual learns to manage his emotions healthily. Consequently, he breaks the link between his emotional life and food, which takes up an appropriate place in his existence: it is the way to satisfy his hunger and not a method to drown his negative emotions in the face of distressing situations. Besides, the meditation and relaxation aspects necessary for hypnosis help the individual to be more aware of his feelings, whether it be his thoughts or his physical state—this can also help to lose weight.

Results After a Session

The success of hypnosis sessions to lose weight goes hand in hand with a solid desire to permanently change bad eating habits.

When the subject is receptive and motivated, he obviously reaches the desired hypnotic state more easily.

After a session, the new behaviors are registered in the subconscious and it becomes easier and natural to stop cracking, to stop giving in to your eating impulses, and to turn to healthy food.

Since a hypnosis session to lose weight is working on the bottom of the problem, the new automatisms are installed in the long term.

Losing those extra pounds is no longer synonymous with stress, frustration, and deprivation. Therapeutic hypnosis helps in particular to maintain its ideal weight and to reach the long-awaited stabilization phase.

Chapter 7:   Meditation and Weight Loss

"Meditation is just hypnosis without a suggestion ..."—most hypnotherapists will tell you that.

And although this may be true in some (very few) cases, it is unfortunate that this opinion is expressed, because it describes only a very limited aspect of meditation and does not take into account the phenomenal number of forms of meditation that exist. It also doesn't take into account the true nature of most forms of meditation.

To illustrate this, I would suggest that you consider the incredible number of guided meditations offered, sold, and promoted by various profit and nonprofit organizations. Of course, to fully understand the implications, one has to consider the composition of most of these guided meditations, which contain some key elements:

1.   Generally designed to create an alternative state of consciousness.

2. Generally designed with a specific life/meditation goal in mind.

3. These goals are sometimes even pursued in the form of a metaphor, whether visualized or not.

4. It can be managed by yourself or by someone else or in a group context with great success.

When you check this, it is clear that there is almost always a goal to be pursued in guided meditations. It must also be recognized that goals cannot be achieved without a proposal to push the specialist in the right direction. Of course, there are various other forms of meditation in which suggestion per se plays a subordinate role. However, it should be noted that meditation without a goal is generally meaningless, and therefore, most forms of meditation are practiced with a specific goal. And it is not surprising that there must also be a proposal in these.

Another example of this would be a simple meditation application for relaxation (a fairly common practice). In this case, a goal remains. "Relaxation." And although the suggestion is generally not passed on during the meditation, it is generally pre-meditation suggestions that are then executed during meditation and generally with the desired results.

So, it would be less than fair to reduce meditation to a meaningless exercise in the definition. Of course, this reminds me of another point of view.

Is there a difference between Hypnosis and meditation? ... After all, they seem to have similar primary properties. And if so, what's the difference, if there is one? ...

Although the answers to these questions are somewhat more complex, it should be noted that while meditation may not be recognized at this point, meditation is a less formalized form of Hypnosis and is considered Hypnosis in most analogies especially when you look at the characteristics of an average meditation.

If you look further at this analogy, you should know that meditation should do the same thing as Hypnosis. It also focuses on creating mental states where the mind can be manipulated to achieve the goals set. One thing to remember, however, is that this is generally practiced in a much less formal setting, and even more in an individual situation that is essentially similar to self-hypnosis. Of course, there are group settings in which meditation is practiced, generally in a guided manner. However, they still retain similar properties and, as such, can be as effective as most forms of Hypnosis practiced.

With this in mind, it seems that there is practically no distinction to be made in the definition except for their use as therapeutic tools.

1. Hypnosis can be used therapeutically to manipulate and control the patient's reactions. This enables direct and immediate adaptable mental therapy in a controlled environment. This also offers therapists the opportunity to treat more severe mental illnesses that meditation would not be suitable for. This is achieved through the creation of external control through Hypnosis that promotes the safe mental healing of patients with fairly serious illnesses. This also offers a fairly simple alternative to meditation for those who do not have the inner ability and strength to hypnotize/meditate on themselves.

2. Meditation can also be used as a therapeutic tool but requires more practitioners' internal skills.

Given the nature of meditation and the significant similarities between meditation and Hypnosis, meditation can be used as efficiently as most self-hypnosis techniques and even some therapeutic uses such as regression and other forms. Advanced meditators are available from related hypnotherapy. A professional can achieve results similar to that of hypnotherapy with meditation, for example, when he says: "Help you quit smoking."

If I accept this, I would suggest that meditators are not afraid to explore their minds and abilities using meditation as a platform and to expand them to what is traditionally considered self-hypnosis techniques. If you do this carefully, you can achieve much more of your meditation in a much shorter time. Especially when techniques of both genders are combined, when the focus is on internal capacity rather than the traditional hypnosis requirement for external control. Applying this also gives you a unique opportunity to set your own hypnosis/meditation goals, which is usually not possible with hypnotherapists as they generally want to decide what is best for you.

If the therapist can be trusted, it can also bring surprising benefits and may result somewhat faster than expected from attempts of doing it yourself.

Learning to lose weight permanently is not always easy. Long after you reach your weight goal, you either have to maintain or risk landing right where you started. There is something that many people overlook: the value of their prospects. Your attitude and mindset can make a significant contribution to motivation and success. If you want to know how to lose weight permanently, first learn how to properly tackle the task, and be mentally prepared for any obstacle that comes your way.

Think about your goals and skills. No, you won't sound crazy when you talk to yourself. Sometimes it is helpful to repeat what you want to do, losing weight permanently. Start with this very simple technique: Create a short phrase that you can tell yourself. This should be done in the morning or before bed (or possibly both).

When trying this technique, keep in mind that the words you say make a difference. Avoid words like "I feel" or "I think" and stick to positive and firm words like "I can" and "I will." You need to create a 100% positive and confident message that you will share with yourself. If you're learning to lose weight permanently, you can say something like, "I'm going to lose weight this week" or "I can reach my ideal weight."

Once you've found a short, easy-to-remember phrase that is completely positive, it's time to put it into practice. Repeat the prayer fourteen times at set times (either before bed or when you wake up). Fourteen works well because there are enough repetitions to keep the thought in your head, but not enough to sound monotonous. The key is to say every word and be serious! You don't have to look in the mirror or anything, just say the sentence orally so I can hear and say it at the same time.

By learning how to lose weight permanently, you are always helping to implement a range of motivational tools to ensure success. If your mind is in the right place, your body will follow you. Try to think of something personal and tangible to remind you of your goals and efforts. For example, while you're at work, you can buy a plate. The reflective type to be used in houses works well because they are larger and more distinctive.

Pick the number that corresponds to the number of pounds you want to lose in a week. Using stickers to indicate your target weight is not recommended in case someone else sees them. Place the sticker where you can easily find it. These motivational tips can help you lose weight permanently if you use Hypnosis or hypnotherapy so you can live a healthier life!

Chapter 8: Strategies for Weight Loss with Hypnosis

Maintaining Mental Strength

Managing stress is the most frequent cause of overeating. Regardless of whether you are aware or not, the chance is to make a fuss because you are worried about other aspects of your life, such as work, personal relationships, and the health of loved ones.

The easiest way to reduce compulsive intake is to manage life stress. This is a solution that cannot be achieved with a tip bag that can help with stressful situations.

Activities such as yoga, meditation, long walks, listening to jazz and classical music can be enjoyed comfortably. Do what you have to do to feel that you are in control of your life. Try to go to bed at the same time every day and get enough rest. If you are well-rested, you will be better able to cope with stressful situations.

Connect Your Mind and Body Over Time

You can get more out of your feelings by writing a diary that lets you write what you have come up with, talk about your desires, and look back after an overwhelming episode.

Taking a little time a day to think about your actions and feelings can have a huge impact on how you approach your life.

Be honest with yourself. Write about how you feel about every aspect of life and your relationship with food.

You can surprise yourself too. You can keep a record of the food you eat unless you are obsessed with every little thing you eat. Sometimes you can escape temptation if you know that you have to write everything you eat.

Take Time to Listen to The Body and Connect it to the Mind

If you know what your body is really telling you, it will be easier for you to understand what will bring you anger and manage your diet. Listen to your body throughout the day and give it time to have a better idea about what it really needs or wants.

Follow the 10-minute rule before eating a snack. If you have a desire, do not grant yourself immediately, wait 10 minutes, and look back at what is actually happening. Ask yourself whether you are hungry or craving. If you are hungry, you have to eat something before your desire grows.

If you have a strong desire but are tired, you must find a way to deal with that feeling. For example, take a walk or do something else to distract yourself from your desires. Ask yourself whether you are eating just because you are bored.

Are you looking in the fridge just because you are looking for something? In that case, find a way to keep yourself active by drinking a glass of water. Please have fun from time to time.

If you have the all-purpose desire to eat peanut butter, eat a spoonful of butter with a banana. This will allow you to reach the bottom after five days and not eat the entire peanut butter jar.

Maintain healthy habits, Eat healthy meals three times a day. This is the easiest way to avoid overeating. If you haven't eaten for half a day, you'll enjoy the fuss. The important thing is to find a way to eat the healthy food you like.

So instead of eating what you really want, you feel that you are fulfilling your duty through a dull and tasteless meal, your meal should be nutritious and delicious.

Follow this method:

Always eat in the kitchen or another designated location. Do not eat even in front of a TV or computer or even when you are on the phone. There is less opportunity to enjoy without concentrating on what you eat. Eat at least 20-25 minutes with each meal.

This may seem like a long time, but it prevents you from feeling when your body is really full. There is a gap between the moment your body is really full and the moment you feel full, so if you bite a bit more time, you will be more aware of how much you eat.

Each meal needs a beginning and an end. Do not bob for 20 minutes while you cook dinner. Also, do not eat snacks while making healthy snacks. You need to eat three types of food, but you should avoid snacking between meals, avoiding healthy options such as fruits, nuts, and vegetables.

Eat meals and snacks in small dishes using small forks and spoons. Small dishes and bowls make you feel as if you are eating more food, and small forks and spoons give you more time to digest the food.

Managing Social Meals

When eating out, it is natural to increase the tendency to loosen up because you feel less controlled than in the normal environment and normal diet options. However, being outside should not be an excuse to enjoy overeating.

You must also find ways to avoid them, even if you are in a social environment or surrounded by delicious food. Follow this method:

Snack before departure. By eating half of the fruit and soup, you can reduce your appetite when surrounded by food. If you are in an area with unlimited snacks, close your hands.

Hold a cup or a small plate of vegetables to avoid eating other foods. If you are in a restaurant, check the menu for healthier options. Try not to be influenced by your friends. Also, if you have a big problem with bread consumption, learn to say "Don't add bread" or have peppermint candy until you have a meal.

Avoid Temptation

Another way to avoid overeating is to stay away from situations that can lead to doing it. Taking steps to avoid overeating when you leave home has a significant impact on how you handle your cravings. This is what you should do:

Try to spend more time on social activities that don't involve eating. Take a walk or walk with friends, or meet friends at a bar that you know is not serving meals. If you are going to a family party that you know will be full of delicious food and desserts, choose a low calorie or healthy option.

Try to escape from unhealthy food when you are at a party. Modify the routine as needed. Eliminate or save a little bit of unhealthy food at home. I don't want to remove all unhealthy snacks from home and go to the stores where they sell at midnight.

Perform an Exercise Routine That You Like

Exercise not only will make you feel healthier, but it will also improve your mental health and make you feel more in control of your body. The trick to exercise is to do something you really like instead of feeling that you are exercising to compensate for binge eating.

Exercise should feel like fun, not torture. Do not do anything you hate. If you hate running, walking or hiking, look for a new activity, such as salsa dancing, Pilates or volleyball. You will have fun doing something you really like and you will get more health in the process. Find a gym or exercise with a friend. Having a friend who works with you will make your training more fun and make you feel more motivated.

Tips

Do not diet. Most likely, dieting will make you feel restricted and consumed by your cravings. Instead, focus on maintaining a healthy lifestyle.

First, consume healthier foods. If you are at a party, start with some healthy entrees, which will slow your appetite and make you less likely to enjoy less healthy foods later. Never eat standing up. Take your time to sit down to eat and focus on food.

Control the portions. Never eat anything from inside a bag or box or you will not know how much you are eating.

Chapter 9:   Creating your Healthy Mindset

Weight loss can appear to be a daunting struggle, utilizing weight loss affirmations to help you in the process can make it simpler. We should feel free to audit this monstrous rundown to assist you with your weight loss venture.

1.   Shedding pounds falls into place without a hitch for me.

2.   I am joyfully accomplishing my weight misfortune objectives.

3.   I am shedding pounds each day.

4.   I love to practice consistently.

5.   I am eating nourishments that adds to my wellbeing and prosperity.

6.   I eat just when I am ravenous.

7.   I presently, obviously observe myself at my optimal weight.

8.   I love the flavor of solid nourishment.

9.   I am in charge of the amount I eat.

10.   I am getting a charge out of working out; it makes me feel great.

11.   I am turning out to be fitter and more grounded regularly through exercise.

12.   I am effectively reaching and keeping up my optimal weight.

13.   I love and care for my body.

14.   I have the right to have a thin, sound, alluring body.

15.   I am growing progressively smart dieting propensities constantly.

16.   I am getting slimmer consistently.

17.   I look and feel incredible.

18.   I take the necessary steps to be sound.

19.   I am joyfully re-imagining achievement.

20.   I decide to work out.

21.   I need to eat foods that cause me to look and to feel great.

22.   I am liable for my wellbeing.

23.   I love my body.

24.   I understand with making my better body.

25.   I am cheerfully practicing each morning when I wake up so I can arrive at the weight loss that I need.

26.   I am subscribing to my weight loss program by changing my dietary patterns from unhealthy to the whole.

27.   I am content with each part I do in my extraordinary exertion to lose weight.

28.   I am consistently getting slimmer and more advantageous.

29.   I am building up an appealing body.

30.   I am building up a way of life of energetic wellbeing.

31.   I am making a body that I like and appreciate.

32.   Positive Affirmations for Losing Weight

33.   The changes in my eating habits are changing my body.

34.   I am feeling incredible since I have lost more than 10 pounds in about a month and can hardly wait to meet my woman companion.

35.   I have a level stomach.

36.   I control my capacity to settle on decisions about food.

37.   I am joyfully gauging 20 pounds less.

38.   I am cherishing strolling 3 to 4 times each week and do conditioning practices, at any rate, three times each week.

39.   I drink eight glasses of water daily.

40.   I eat leafy foods day by day and eat, for the most part, chicken and fish.

41.   I am learning and utilizing the psychological, passionate, and otherworldly aptitudes for progress. I will change it!

42.   I will make new contemplations about myself and my body.

43.   I cherish and value my body.

44.   It's energizing to find my exceptional nourishment and exercise framework for weight loss.

45.   I am a weight loss example of overcoming adversity.

46.   I am charmed to be the perfect weight for me.

47.   It's simple for me to follow a whole foods plan.

48.   I decided to grasp the contemplations of trust in my capacity to roll out positive improvements throughout my life.

49.   It feels great to move my body. Exercise is enjoyable!

50.   I utilize profound breathing to assist me with unwinding and handle the pressure.

51.   I am a delightful individual.

52.   I have the right to be at my optimal weight.

53.   I am an adorable individual. I merit love. It is OK for me to lose weight.

54.   I am really close to reaching my lower weight.

55.   I lose the need to reprimand my body.

56.   I acknowledge and make the most of my sexuality. It's OK to feel exotic.

57.   My digestion is incredible.

58.   I keep up my body with ideal wellbeing.

These weight loss affirmations will assist you with making your way towards getting thinner. I trust these 50 weight loss affirmations proved to be useful. Try to bookmark this page for future reference.

Positive Affirmations for Stress Reduction

Encountering a specific level of worry in life is inescapable. In any case, feelings of anxiety that stay high more often than not can effectively affect an individual's physical and passionate prosperity.

Discovering approaches to oversee pressure is primary for acceptable wellbeing and bliss, and repeating positive affirmations is a useful method to expand sentiments of internal harmony. The ongoing examination has presumed that positive affirmations can support against the impacts of pressure and increment an individual's critical thinking capacity and errand execution (J. David Creswell, 2013). Positive affirmations are engaging explanations that you repeat to yourself with certainty. These announcements assist you with imagining and cement in your brain how you need to respond and feel in specific circumstances or by and large. They are spoken in the current state and mirror the things you need to find in your life.

Positive affirmations, repeated to yourself with power, can help increment your certainty and conviction that you can deal with life well and receive all that you need in return. They can achieve a diminished feeling of anxiety, a more settled mentality, and better wellbeing.

How Do Positive Affirmations Work?

In case you're thinking, "It appears to be unrealistic that conversing with myself can completely change me," how about we consider it like this: when we feel and carry on positively, life appears to go all the more easily. At the point when we are feeling negative about ourselves, irritable, and opposite, things look to go ineffectively. We may take part in foolish practices that cause things to go severely. Interminable pressure and antagonism can even prompt medical issues.

As such, our considerations impact our activities, which influence our conditions.

Positive affirmations are said in the current state. This is somewhat hard for specific individuals because the statement might be something they don't feel directly at that point. The key is to prepare your brain to accept the announcement through reiteration and, in this way, start to feel the sentiments related to the report. At the point when that occurs, you will be bound to take the activities that are important to accomplish that positive change. Here are two models:

You need to lose some weight. You utilize the affirmation, "I am sound and delightful." Feeling alluring and fit causes you to feel great and encourages you to participate in more fixed schedules as opposed to enjoying wellbeing undermining ones out of the requirement for comfort. The welfare transforms you're after, for example, weight loss, will happen more effectively than they would if you reveal to yourself something more along the lines of "I will feel delightful after I lose 10 pounds."

You need to get another line of work, and you have a meeting. You utilize the affirmation, "I am equipped for this position, and the questioner sees my worth." Going into the meeting, faith in this affirmation permits you to act normally and positively. If you by some means happened to state to yourself, "I trust I land this position! I would prefer not to wreck this meeting," stress could lead you to carry on contrastingly in the meeting, likely more apprehensively and with less certainty; less ready to flaunt your aptitudes.

As should be obvious, utilizing positive affirmations to change your idea, examples and desires can pull in positive outcomes into your life.

How Might You Make Positive Affirmations Work the Best for You?

There are a few things you can improve to the intensity of positive affirmations in diminishing your feelings of anxiety and expanding your adapting capacities.

Pick a positive affirmation that speaks to the musings, sentiments, or good life that you wish to have. You could likewise keep in touch with one (or many) yourself.

Repeat the positive affirmation to yourself a few times in succession a couple of times each day. Redundancy can help offer the expression increasingly concrete in your brain.

Inhale profoundly multiple times in succession before starting your recitation of the affirmation. Concentrate your psyche on the words that you're repeating as opposed to what's happening around you.

Repeat the affirmation to yourself on occasion when your brain is usually increasingly loosened up, for example, just after waking or as you're nodding off. It tends to be extra fantastic to repeat positive affirmation delicately as you nod off.

Positive Affirmations to Release Stress

Alongside day by day positive affirmations to buy and significant increment the inspiration in your life, here are some incredible statements that can explicitly assist you with discharging pressure immediately when you feel overpowered. Take a couple of seconds for yourself to inhale profoundly and repeat one of these affirmations a couple of times. Envision yourself, discharging the pressure from your psyche and the strain from your body with each breathes out. Here are a couple of affirmations from which you can pick:

1.   I am glad, quiet, and liberated from stress.

2.   I am a positive individual who pulls in positive things into my life.

3.   I am prepared to deal with this circumstance successfully.

4.   My body and psyche feel quiet and tranquil.

5.   Useful things persistently transpire.

6.   I radiate a feeling of prosperity and cause others in my quality to feel good and great about themselves.

7.   Feeling loose is my normal state.

8.   I feel without a care in the world since it's useful for my wellbeing.

9.   I am in charge of my life and decide to feel quiet.

10.   I am sure about my life and my capacities.

11.   I forgive myself for the missteps I have made previously, and I have gained from them.

12.   There are a few things I can't change, and I'm OK with that.

13.   I decide to discharge sentiments of stress and grasp blissful considerations.

14.   This circumstance will pass, so I decide to manage it smoothly.

15.   I consider difficulties to be life exercises for me to find out more and be a superior individual.

16.   I am a decent individual who merits satisfaction, wellbeing, and harmony.

The more you repeat these affirmations to yourself, the more rapidly and viably they will assist you with discharging pressure when required.

Chapter 10: How to Maintain Eating Habits in Your Life

If you think that what I prescribe is just a diet, you've got it wrong. Experts have long said that to keep weight off, people need to make long-term changes to their diet and activity levels. According to the CDC, those who lose weight at a pace of one to two pounds per week tend to keep weight off more successfully. Further, they emphasize how important it is to take steps to ensure you maintain your weight loss.

Hypnosis is different from normal "diets" because it doesn't promote temporary change. Hypnotherapy helps you resist going back to your old ways, but that doesn't mean that you don't also need to keep up your efforts. Hypnosis instills a tendency towards long term change, but if you don't fight to keep that change up, you're going to go back to how you were. Accordingly, take the messages you learn through hypnosis and reinforce them as much as you can after you've finished hypnotherapy. You can continue to use scripts on your own if you want to ensure that you maintain progress.

Too many people return to their original weights after they lose weight. Only about ten to twenty percent of people keep weight off and don't return to their original weight or higher after losing weight. This weight is often regained within five years, sometimes in as little time as just weeks, depending on how much you've lost. Thus, if you don't remain conscious of your habits, you may start to incorporate the ones that you'd ditched.

Carry all the changes you've made through even after you've stopped hypnotherapy. You probably won't want to continue hypnotherapy forever, but you need to keep up with all the dietary, physical, and mental changes that you've made on this journey because they are vital to your overall well-being and happiness. Don't let this journey end by returning to who you were. Continue on your path of growth.

You have to continue fighting for your health, and when you're stressed or anxious, doing this may get hard, but there's no end to maintaining your health. That is something that you'll have to do for the rest of your life. You cannot avoid the effort required to maintain your new weight, but it does get easier over time. You get used to the changes, and the changes eventually feel so natural that they are incredibly easy to keep up.

Don't Forget What You've Fought for

Never forget the effort you put in once you get to your goal weight. You need to remember the time and energy you invested so that you feel motivated not to go back. You don't want to lose your progress and start all over. Thus, never forget that struggle and when you want to return to old habits, remember how long it took you to lose weight and also remember the money you paid to get better (because no one wants to pay more money than they need to!). You don't need to go back, and you have the skills to keep moving forward.

Keep a picture of your old self handy. You can pull this picture out when you need a visual reminder of how far you've come. Remember that older adult and know that you don't want to be them anymore. You've become a person that makes you happier, and there's no need to sabotage the better you. Respect your personal growth by loving the person you were without wanting to be that person anymore. You were fine just as you were in the past, but your changed self feels better, and that's the difference.

Remember how bad you felt before you made a change. You wanted to change for a reason! You weren't comfortable in your skin before you made the change, so you need never to forget that you changed for a reason. You wanted to grow as a person, and you accomplished this goal by dreaming of a better self and working to make that person a reality.

Think of how much better you feel now that you've made a change. Doesn't it feel exhilarating to take an issue and watch as it gradually improves? Of course, it does, so take that victorious feeling and carry it with you whenever temptation may strike. When you want to eat a whole bag of chips, think of how much better you'd feel if you didn't do that.

Promise yourself that you're never going to go backward. Repeat this message to yourself every day if you need to because if you tell yourself that it won't happen, your brain is likely to listen. You have to keep going forward, or you'll end up running in dissatisfying circles. It can be so easy to get stuck in the past and let everything that allured you into a false sense of security, but by relying so much on the past, you will lose sight of the present, and you will forfeit much of the happiness you could have by not seeing all the beautiful things that are right there in front of you.

Know that the future is yours for the taking. You decide what you want your future to be, and you build it. There are some variables in life that you have no power over, and those things can be terrifying and make you not want to think about the future. You get hurt, people die, you change jobs, etc. A lot will change in the future in ways you can't predict, but you have the power to take those changes positively or negatively. Any change can be used to better yourself in some way. You just have to determine how you will use that change to your advantage.

Choose healthy choices. Once you've lost weight, you are not permitted to stop eating nutrient-dense foods. Your body still needs fruits, vegetables, healthy fats, proteins, and whole grains just as much as it did before. Don't start turning to foods with empty calories for meals. Continue to cook well-balanced meals and eat foods that are good for your body, and that will give you the energy you need to carry you through the day.

Always tend to your emotional and physical needs. These needs should come before anything else. Prioritize what your body wants from you and let your body be cherished instead of degraded. Attending to your needs signals to your body that you are taking care of it, which will reduce your cravings for certain foods and unhealthy behaviors that have haunted you in the past. Continue to practice mindful eating and remain aware of your emotions to ensure that you don't neglect your body or mind.

You've worked so hard to make progress, so it would make you feel like the worst person alive to go back on those changes once you've finally reached your weight-loss goal. Accordingly, you need to keep reminding yourself of how far you've come so that the victory of your weight loss is always fresh in your mind. Feel proud of your progress, proud enough that you hold yourself accountable to keep up that progress even when it is hard to do so (because some days will be harder than others).

Stay Active

Humans need activity. It's important to keep doing things and accomplishing physical feats even if you've already met your goal weight. Once you've lost weight, you may be able to ease up on the activity, but it will hurt your physical and emotional health to quit being active altogether. Boredom is one of the biggest reasons people overeat, so keep yourself busy to avoid the pitfalls of having nothing to do but to eat as you watch TV.

Continue your physical activity. If you've found physical activities that you love, don't quit them once you've reached your goal weight. Continue to let them better your life and drive you to be a happier and healthier person. Stay in tune with your body's needs and find power in all the wonderful things your body can do.

Challenge the activity you already do and try to keep pushing yourself. I bet that you can be doing more than you are. Don't let your workout regime become stagnant. Keep pushing your skills and building your body up. You should never be content with how you are right now. You can always do more and improve your physical condition.

Maintain hobbies that bring your fulfillment. Studies have shown that hobbies are good for your health and to reduce stress. These hobbies don't have to be physical, but keeping hobbies will give you purpose, and projects help keep you motivated. You need to have outlets for your creative energy, which can be found through hobbies. Your hobbies should be recreational and have nothing to do with your work or other responsibilities. Hobbies such as constructing models, writing, or drawing are all just a few ideal options for people to consider. Some of the most common hobbies are games, collecting things, outdoor activity, or building things. The possibilities are endless!

Be mentally active. Finding pursuits that challenge your brain can be a strong way to keep yourself occupied. Maybe you like to complete puzzles. Maybe you like to write stories. Maybe you like to solve riddles. Maybe you like to read books. Whatever it is that keeps your mind active, do it. Your brain is a muscle, and you can train it just as you can other parts of your body, so don't neglect your brain. It will get bored if you don't keep it on its toes!

Spend time with people who make you feel good about yourself. Maintain quality friendships once you have lost weight. Don't find people who only accept you because you have lost weight or who will make you feel bad about yourself. Choose to spend your time with people who will keep you engaged in your relationships and feeling confident about those friendships. Supportive people are just as important when you maintain your weight as when you lose weight.

Being active is one of the best ways to maintain your weight, and it doesn't matter what methods you choose to keep you busy, but try to maintain several things that keep you staying strong and reaching for opportunities that make you happy and secure in your position in life. Being active will help you keep bad habits out.

Chapter 11:   How to Use Hypnosis for Change in Eating Habits

It's impractical for any of us to believe we should be conscious of every bite or even of every meal we consume. The demands of work and family often imply that you're expected to feed on the run or have just a short window for the remainder of the day to feed something or face starvation. But even though you can't stick to a rigorous practice of mindful feeding, you can also resist mindless eating and following the body's warnings. Before consuming a meal or snack, maybe you should take a few deep breaths and silently consider what you will bring into your stomach. In reaction to hunger cues, are you feeding, or are you feeding in reaction to an emotional signal? Are you bored or nervous or lonely, perhaps?

Similarly, are you consuming nutritionally balanced food, or are you consuming mentally comforting food? Even though, for example, you have to feed at your workplace, will you take a couple of minutes instead of multitasking or getting interrupted by your screen or phone to concentrate all your energy on your food? Think of mindful eating as an exercise: it counts every little bit.

The more you will do to calm down, reflect solely on the feeding process, and respond to your body, the greater enjoyment you can feel from your meals and the more influence you can have regarding your diet and dietary behaviors.

Exploring your Relationship with Food Using Mindfulness

Food dramatically affects your well-being, whether you are aware of it or not. The way you feel physically, react emotionally, and cope mentally may be influenced. It can improve your energy and perspective, or it can drain your assets and render you feel tired, moody, and discouraged.

We all agree that sugar, refined foods, and more berries and vegetables can be consumed. Because if it were necessary to recognize the "laws" of safe living, neither of us would be overweight or hooked on fast food. However, once you eat deliberately and become more attuned to the body, you will begin to feel how various foods physically, psychologically, and emotionally impact you. And it will make the transition to better eating options far simpler to make.

For starters, if you know that when you're exhausted or stressed, the candy snack you want simply leaves you feeling much worse, it's better to control those cravings and just go for a healthy snack that improves your energy and mood.

When it allows us to be mentally sick, we always focus on how food makes us act. The query that we need to address is not, "Does my diet make me sick?" But rather, "How nice is it going to make me feel?" How much healthier do you feel after eating, in other words? After a meal or snack, how much more energy and excitement do you have?

How Does Your Food Make You Feel?

It's important to become conscious of how various foods make you truly discover your relationship with food. How do you feel after five minutes, an hour, or a few hours of eating? How are you usually doing during the day? Try the following experiment to begin to observe the relationship between what you consume and how it makes you feel:

Tracking the Link Between Food and Feeling

Regularly, eat. Choose the ingredients, quantities, and periods you usually consume, but now emphasize what you do. Keep a list during meals of everything things you consume, like snacks and treats. Don't fool yourself; whether you type it all down or track it in an app, you won't recall it all. Give attention to the physical and mental emotions five minutes after waking, one hour after eating, two or three hours after eating.

Note whether a shift or transition has arisen because of eating. Are you doing better or worse than you did before eating? Are you feeling energized or weary? Alert or dull? Keeping a record on your mobile or in a journal can improve your understanding of how your mood and well-being are influenced by the meals and snacks you eat.

Experimenting with Different Food Combinations

The method of eating food becomes a practice of listening to your own body until you can relate your food preferences to your mental and physical well-being. For instance, you might notice that you look sluggish and lethargic for hours after you consume carbohydrates. Carb-heavy foods, then, is something that you try to prevent. Of course, due to influences such as genetics and lifestyle, multiple foods impact us all differently. So, finding the foods and variations of food that work best for you can require some trial and error. The following exercise will help you learn how multiple food combinations and quantities influence your well-being:

Mixing and Matching Different Foods

Start experimenting with your food:

- Start consuming fewer things more frequently, or fewer meals, ever.

- Spend two to three days removing meat from your diet, whether you are a meat-eater.

- Or maybe you should remove red meat, but you should add poultry and fish.

- Delete from your diet these foods: salt, caffeine, sugar, or pizza, for instance, to see if this influence if you feel.

- Play with combinations of foods. Aim to consume carbohydrate meals, protein, meat, or vegetable meals only.

- Keep a note when you play in your dietary patterns with everything that you notice in yourself. The query you are seeking to address is: "Which eating habits lead to the value of my life, and what diverts attention from that?" For two to three weeks, begin playing with multiple styles, ratios, and quantities of food, monitoring how psychologically, physically, and emotionally you feel.

Eating to Fill a Void vs. Eating to Improve Well-being

Although food undeniably influences how you feel, it's still quite true that when, where, and how much you consume affects how you feel. Many of us sometimes confuse feelings of fear, fatigue, isolation, or frustration for hunger pangs and use food to deal with these emotions. The pain you experience tells you that you desire more and need something in your life to fill a void. A stronger friendship, a more rewarding career, or a spiritual desire might be the need. However, as you continuously want to fill gaps with food, you eventually forget your true hunger.

You will become conscious of how much your food intake has little to do with actual hunger and all to do with satisfying an emotional desire while practicing mindful eating, and your knowledge increases. When you sit down and feed, question yourself, "What am I hungry for?" Since you're very hungry or for some excuse, are you wanting the "tiny bit to nibble on"?

Filling yourself with food and saturating yourself will help hide what you're starving for, but just for a little while. And then the true starvation or need would come back. Practicing mindful eating helps you calm down, reflect on the actual moment, and understand what you truly thought. And when you question yourself frequently, "After a meal or snack, how well do I feel?" The phase of acquiring knowledge of your dietary requirements will start.

Taking Deep Breaths Before You Eat

Breathing can also help alleviate hunger, particularly when food often isn't about hunger. Oxygen fuels our body, and the energy and feeling of well-being will be enhanced by breathing deeply. You also ease stress and tension, typical copycats of false hunger, when you breathe deeply.

8 Mindful Habits You Practice Everyday

1. Sit in the morning

A fantastic chance to practice mindfulness is offered in the morning. The day is just starting, it's quiet and nice, and you may have a few memories to yourself. I enjoy waiting for a couple of minutes instead of jumping out of bed and going through the morning routine. I'm just speaking of being happy for the day and making myself be in the moment. You may only want to relax on the sofa and focus on synchronized breathing, or meditation may also take place. I notice that doing so allows me to begin with the correct mind frame every day.

2. Eat Mindfully

What was the last moment you enjoyed a meal? That's easily understandable. Your life is complicated, and as a result, eating has been something accomplished in passing. We have fast-food chains that we can also travel around and consume while we travel. Alternatively, I encourage you to try to slow down, make food for yourself, and eat deliberately.

Choose live foods with a selection of shades, textures, and tastes that are different. Take the time to truly chew each bite and enjoy it. For digestion, doing so is healthier and can be a fun and calming period. So many of us carry distractions to the table as an extra point. Some people watch TV, others learn, and others may not be able to put down their mobile.

3. Spend Time Outside

Another approach to obtain mindfulness would be to invest a little time outside, and you don't need to head to a far-off resort to achieve the optimal effects. Everything you need to do is go for a stroll in your neighborhood. They will make the ideal place to stay in contact with nature and interact with the current moment, whether you have beautiful paths, parks, or green areas. Watch what you see on your hike, how you feel about the weather, what you listen to, and what smell.

4. Meditate

The art of mindfulness is meditation. You take the opportunity to engage with your mind when meditating. It requires some time to learn controlled breathing and quiet out all the noise, but it can be useful in many respects. It may also be useful for relaxing and stress management and being a period for mindfulness.

5. Focus on One Task at a Time

It is almost natural to assume that achieving everything at once is easier, but it is not real. You do not give each of them the attention they need by splitting the energy into several activities. Studies also show that multitasking raises the probability of errors as it takes longer than completing the activities individually. Taking one job at a time and concentrate on the mission at hand. Take a quick break when you are finished and then pursue the next mission. It is a more comfortable and aware way to get stuff accomplished, and the efficiency would hopefully increase.

6. Feel Feelings

You must not avoid your feelings during being mindful. In the current moment, part of life is exactly the way it is. It may involve excitement at times, but you don't want to continue to push positive emotions or avoid some real emotional reaction. Perhaps, because of the moment, you only need to recognize negative feelings. Accept dishonesty, jealousy, sorrow, frustration, etc. as what they are and enable yourself to feel them. You ought to be aware of how you react to emotions but accepting them for what they are is safe.

7. Create Something

This will also be a successful way to exercise mindfulness if you have an artistic hobby. Your artistic side is mindful of its essence, whether you want to sketch, paint, create, or take photographs. The practice of mindfulness, as a bonus, will inspire imagination. You may notice that fresh and innovative thoughts come to you more quickly while you are on a stroll or meditating.

8. Engage in Physical Activities You are Passionate About

When we do something we love and which needs the body and mind's concentration, it is easiest to be mindful. Surfing, basketball, soccer, or cycling, for instance. It can mean a missing target or be tossed about in a breaking wave if you forget your mindfulness when participating in these practices. You can spend time fully engaged by finding an activity you enjoy that can teach you how to bring that mindfulness into other aspects of life. You will feel that you have achieved a different type of power over your life because you are more mindful and in the moment. It's going to help you achieve an overall satisfaction that's not that temporary. Check out any of these strategies to see the difference mindfulness can create.

Chapter 12: Using Hypnosis to Change Eating Habits

Pay Attention to Your Habits

Habits rule much of your everyday activities, especially your food and exercise habits. In addition to hypnosis, paying attention to your habits is an important step in weight loss because it's your habits that dictate whether you will adapt your eating habits to match what goals you need to make. Forty percent of what you do each day is habitual, so if you don't pay attention to your habits, you're missing an important chunk of your behavior and failing to make it align with your goals. If you want to lose weight some, but not all, habits will have to change.

Because so much of our life is ruled by habits, you need to determine what your worst dietary and exercise habits are. For one week or so, keep track of your eating and exercise patterns, especially pay attention to times when you mindlessly eat or emotionally eat. Track what you eat and why you are eating it. Also, track the kinds of exercises you do and for how long. During this process, you can begin to pick up on some of your habits that may not be initially apparent when you try to pinpoint the habits you want to change. Some of your habits may be obvious from the start, but others will be more covert. Once you have discovered your habits, find ways to replace your bad habits with good ones to encourage the changes that you want in your life.

91

Replacing unhealthy habits can be hard because habits are so ingrained in you that you often don't notice that you are doing them, but focusing on creating good habits instead of bad ones can brighten your attitude and make it easier to stick to your plan. As you replace your bad habits, create habits that you enjoy and that give you enrichment. If you don't like celery, don't replace your chip eating habit with a celery eating habit. Try carrots and hummus or rice cakes. There are hundreds of good alternatives to anyone bad habit, so find ones that work for you and don't make you feel like you're completely losing.

Don't try to change everything at once. Start one or a couple of habits at a time. If you try to do too much habit-changing at once, your brain will struggle to focus and keep up with all the changes that you need to be making. Integrate your new habits gradually, so that it's not a shock to your system. You have plenty of time to complete your transformation, so don't rush it. You wouldn't want a contractor rushing to build your house just to get it done, and you'd be angry if he did a half-hearted job, so you need to take your time with your weight loss and do it the proper and effective way. If you can manage to break more than a couple of habits at once, throw in some more habits to break, but as always, know your limits.

Reward yourself when you do well. Encourage yourself whenever you find yourself not doing your bad habits. For example, if you're able to make it twenty-one days without mindlessly eating in front of the TV, promise yourself that you can go get your nails done or that you can buy a pair of new shoes. Make it worth your while. Giving yourself things to look forward to is a huge motivation and puts your mind on what you can gain instead of letting it fixate on what you're losing. It may be hard to see this now, but by the end of your journey, you won't feel like you've lost anything. You'll merely feel balanced, and like you've gained a new chance to be the person you want to be.

Get your loved ones involved in your weight loss journey and allow them to be part of your plans. Maybe one of your friends also wants to lose weight or achieve new fitness goals. Going on this journey together can be an important bonding experience, and not having to go through the process alone makes it significantly easier. So, if you find a friend who is willing and able, be each other's support system and hold each other accountable. Even if they don't diet with you, lean on your family and friends to be your cheerleaders, and push you to be your best self even when you are feeling discouraged.

Get rid of things that might encourage bad habits. If you're a chip junkie, limit how many chips you keep in your house. When you have habits that you want to get rid of, the best thing you can do is to keep the temptations far away. That way, when you'd normally habitually reach for the bag of chips, you have to consciously become aware of the fact that you don't have any chips. From there, you are given a decision to either teach yourself to reach for something else, or you have to consciously go out of your way to get those chips. When you have to consciously do something, that's helping you resist the habitual draw because you have to stop and think about what you are doing.

Use visualization to see yourself as the person you want to be. Visualization is a superb tool to help you imagine your goals and then achieve them. Imagine yourself where you want to be one year from now. Think of how you'll look, but also imagine how you will feel. Think of how you'll move differently when you lose weight. Think of all the obstacles you'll no longer have to face. Think of the freedom you will feel and the weight that will be lifted from your shoulders. Imagine yourself as calm, stress-free, and thinner. Each day, it can help to go to bed and wake up, visualizing the person you'd like to be.

Be aware of the hardship and the payoff. Always keep the payoff in your mind and remind yourself why you want to change. If you don't keep what you want in the forefront of your mind, your dreams will get lost in the chaos of your head. The hardship seems a lot worse when you think of all the amazing things that can come from that work. Challenges can also be psychologically rewarding because, when you don't feel challenged, you feel bored and stagnated, which leads to restlessness and unhappiness.

Don't allow yourself to say that it's not working and give up. Be patient with yourself. If you're only a week in, and you're already starting to convince yourself that it's hopeless, then you're the problem. When you don't let yourself see the whole process through, you are failing yourself, and you are refusing to accomplish the steps you need to take to become the person you want to be. Go back and do more mental preparation until you feel ready to give this your all. Give yourself at least a month. Habits can take anywhere from twenty-one days up to two months to form. Thus, if you don't stick that time out, don't give up on your dieting plans until you've at least given a one-month effort, preferably more. If you give it that long, you'll find that it starts to get easier

Start right away. Don't put weight loss off until tomorrow. You need to start this process right now and not let yourself run away fearfully from the things that you want to accomplish. If you don't start right away, you will keep putting your weight-loss dreams off until there isn't another tomorrow. There's absolutely no reason to delay this journey. It may seem overwhelming now, but it's completely manageable for anyone willing to put the time and effort in.

Set Yourself Up for Success

The ultimate goal of hypnosis and the heart of this whole book is to set yourself up for success. So many diets are bound to fail, but because this plan allows you to make permanent changes and to teach your brain to act in better ways, accordingly, you aren't set up to fail. Though, as good as this information is, the brunt of the burden of success is on you. You're the one who has to put in all the work to set yourself up for success, so take that duty seriously.

Take the time to focus on yourself. It's not selfish to want to take some special time to care for your own needs. So many people dedicated their lives to other people, and that's a noble thing, but every person also needs to care for their own needs so that they can better serve other people and feel confident about who they are. Find time to reflect on your growth and weight-loss journey in addition to finding time for hypnosis. We all have busy lives, but cutting back on one TV episode a day can make an immense difference in how much you can accomplish. You deserve to feel good about yourself, so prioritize that, and you'll be able to find the time.

Be open to change. You're not going to be able to stick by your old and comfortable habits. You'll have to learn to welcome in the new and embrace the uncertainty that every new journey brings. Sometimes you will feel like you're so far out of your element, but that's a good thing! When you feel like that, you are changing and growing as a person. Don't be afraid to try new things and experiment with what you eat and what activities you do. There's no limit to how much you can learn about yourself, and of course, if you're open to change, you'll welcome the weight loss. Too many people subconsciously close themselves off to weight loss, so make a conscious effort to remain open to new information about the world and yourself.

Don't doubt yourself. Have faith in your ability to accomplish your goals. There's genuinely nothing to stand in your way of success. You hold all the power in this transformation, so if you want to do well, believing in yourself can go a long way.

Hypnotherapy can work better when you're in the right headspace to do it, which is why we have emphasized getting into the right headspace for hypnosis and learning about what hypnosis fundamentally is. With all the information you've read so far, you should feel ready to set yourself up for success and finally dive into the actual hypnosis. There will still be plenty of mental work ahead, but now that you've created the mental foundation, you can handle all of it with grace and relative ease. Your mind has amazing powers, ones you only need to channel to do well. Never question that you can make changes that will last for the rest of your life.

Chapter 13: What is Emotional Eating

Food choices, while in turmoil, can reflect what emotions are causing your desire to eat. The different types of emotional needs like stress, fatigue, or boredom, prompt you to eat different foods.

Knowing the reason behind emotional eating is the first step to conquering it. Pay attention to how you feel when you eat the foods you eat. You will notice the connection between stress and food.

When you're stressed or frustrated, you tend to look for chewy or crunchy foods like cookies or candy bars. When you're feeling sad, lonely, or depressed, you tend to look for soft or creamy textured foods like ice cream or chocolate. Sadness, loneliness, and depression reflect a lack of love and attention.

When you pay attention to the pattern of eating, you will notice the difference between the two types of eating. Once you identify what is leading you to desire to eat, you can take care of what you need instead of looking for it in food.

This is not the blanket one to identify the connection. It may not work for everyone. There are times you won't identify the specific need that you have, but keep searching. Eventually, you will know the exact connection between food and emotions to a certain degree of accuracy.

Pressure Emotions; Anger, Frustration, or Resentment

The cravings are for a specific food. You know exactly what you want. The craving is so precise that you can go to the food store to get a specific brand of cookies or nuts. You do what it takes to satisfy the food thought, including getting up in the night to get a bag of French fries.

Foods that you crave when you are frustrated often include nuts, French fries, chewy, meat, hot dogs, pizza or crackers. These foods provide the chewiness or crunchiness that requires an effort to give the feeling of satisfaction. It replaces the thought of having to express frustration or anger to somebody else. Instead, you direct it to food.

The craving for these foods pops up quickly. Within a minute, you are desperately craving for them. Once you finish eating, you feel better for a while. The food soothes the intense emotions that you had, and you feel calmer and peaceful, albeit temporarily. It is good to note down when this happens so that you can work on it.

We should eat to provide our body with nourishment and energy. But we eat for many other reasons. We eat the way we do because of our culture and how we were brought up. We eat out of habit or to satisfy expectations from our peers. Other times we eat in response to our emotions, whether to calm down anger or to comfort us. We also eat from compulsion or as a reward.

The primary reason for eating should be to satisfy the physical hunger, which is the body's way of getting the fuel it needs to function throughout the day. In our current fast-paced society, our intake of food is much greater than we need. Our level of activity is nonexistent. Everything has been made easy to achieve. At work, we labor at our desks until dawn. When we get home, the ease of remote-controlled gadgets keeps us on the couch as we watch TV, dim the lights or close the curtains. The result is that we are suffering from the choices that we have made.

To reverse this, we need to create a life of balance. Plan the day in terms of what activities to do and what food to eat. When there is a sense of balance, you can enjoy life. You balance your nutrition, activities, and rest time. Organize your weekly menu plan and your grocery shopping. Schedule all the activities that you need to do at work and home

The Effect of Culture on How We Eat

Our culture determines our relationship with food. It determines how we combine foods and how we eat food. Some cultures embrace vegetarianism, while others eat more animal meats than plant-based diets. Some cultures place importance on sharing meals and eating together.

The cultural norms play a huge role in the relationship that you have with food. List down some food cultures you can remember growing up so that you can discover the relationship you have with food. List how you can still practice your culture without affecting your relationship with food.

Childhood Experiences with Food

As adults, we eat just the same way our parents or guardian taught us. Try to remember what food patterns you learned as a child and how it has impacted your life as an adult.

Some practices include cleaning up your plate. If it was wrong to leave some food on your plate, and you could not leave the dinner table before you finish your food as a child, you will find that as an adult you may overeat so that you don't pour food.

If the practice was to always finish up dinner with a cup of tea or a sweet dessert, you tend to continue with the same in adulthood. What are some of the childhood memories that you have about food? Was it used as a reward or punishment?

Do You Find Yourself Doing These Things As an Adult?

Write down the answer to these questions so that you can trace the connection between your childhood and your current eating patterns and include ways you can adjust.

Comfort Foods

There are foods that you mostly eat when sad or disappointed with what has happened during the day. These foods comfort you. Often you pick them unconsciously, but the truth is, your mind craves them because of the warmth and comfort they make you get.

We can trace some of them back to your childhood. If your parents would make for you chicken soup or hot chocolate to make you feel better, there are high chances that you will use them to comfort you when you're in distress.

The problem is that you have gotten used to using the food for comfort that you don't remember the consequence they could cause like making you gain weight, threaten your health status or even shorten your life expectancy.

Remember that you may feel comforted for some time but still slip back to the feeling of sadness. When we eat these comfort foods often enough in excess amounts, the relationship that we have with food becomes unhealthy. We then feel guilty about the lack of control. This negative feeling then makes us eat some more comfort foods, and the negative cycle continues.

But you can stop the cycle. You need to be aware of the foods that you eat for comfort. Then come up with strategies to counter the need to get food when you are in distress. You can choose to go out for a movie with a friend or get a hot shower or snuggle with your pet instead of eating.

Emotional Eating at Social Events

It is hard to imagine a social gathering without lots of food and drinks, from baptism to church events, to birthdays, graduation parties, and charity events. When we attend such events, we expect to be well fed. So, these social gatherings often have an abundance of food displays of both healthy and unhealthy foods and drinks.

Most People Cannot Turn Down Food When with Friends or Family

You can decide to limit your portions when serving food. Keep chewing gum at hand after you have had your fill to avoid going back for second helpings. You can also brush and floss your teeth so that you don't have an urge to eat. Ask yourself if the food is worth the struggle when your weight goes out of control. Is it worth the struggle to lose it off again?

I know the mind tricks you by telling you that it's just for a day. But imagine if you attend such events once every week. It means that you derail your goals every week. It will be very easy to give up your healthy eating routine if you keep budging in every time you go to social events.

Write down how you can control your food intake at social events. You will need this list to remind you to stay on track and not let one event affect your health goals. Remind yourself that you are in control. You can do this.

Understanding Your Food Habits

You're eating habits is the routine that you are accustomed to in terms of food choices and how much and how often you eat daily. You habitually eat some foods without much thought because it has become your behavior. It could be that you automatically add salt to your food at the table or eat bacon and eggs with toast for breakfast every morning.

List down all the food habits you can think of. Are they healthy?

Using Food For Reward

After a long month of work and no play, you know you deserve a treat. What comes to your mind when you want to treat yourself for a job well done? Is it ice cream or cake? Or do you go to the spa?

You shouldn't always reward yourself with sugary or high-fat food. You could go for dinner to a restaurant that serves healthy whole foods.

Rewards don't need to be just-food. You can treat yourself to food but don't make it a habit. Using food to reward children for good behavior is catastrophic. Children will pick up this habit and continue with this in adulthood. The reason food is what comes to mind when you want to treat yourself could be traced back to your childhood if your parents used pizza or cake or other foods to reward you for good grades or good behavior.

You need to come up with new ideas for rewards or treats yourself or your family. First, note down the foods that you use to reward yourself of your family. Are they healthy foods? What non-food treats can you try?

When you banish the idea that only food can be used for reward, you will gain back your control in terms of your relationship with food. Rewarding yourself for achievement or an important milestone is good.

There are nonfood rewards that you can try, such as a bubble bath, manicure or pedicure, full-body scrub at the spa, travel to your favorite destination. If you can't get time to schedule these ideas, you can come up with other quick rewards that you fancy.

A good idea is choosing a reward that you can do at work, and it can also involve others like your colleagues or family. Just choose what works for you. Write down a few ideas so that you can always refer to the list when you want a treat.

Chapter 14: Causes of Emotional Eating

When it refers to hypnotherapy, individuals have a few choices: One-on-one appointments with a hypnotherapist, listening to tapes of hypnosis, and self-hypnosis. Among the most convenient ones is self-hypnosis, so you can do it in the warmth of your own house or at the workplace.

For compulsive eating, it is often strongly advised. The method is, as you can see, easy. Here are some aspects you may like to remember:

Consider Your Well-Being—How do you feel? Evaluating how you felt is beneficial because, by the conclusion of the session, you can reevaluate it.

Directed Breathing & Visualization—The body and mind acquire deep breathing as a message that it is time to rest. Another strategy for triggering relaxation is imagination.

A Directed Countdown—From 10, you can choose to countdown. This allows the brain to move into a hypnosis mode.

Strong Affirmations—You should talk explicitly to the subconscious when you're comfortable. Give it affirmations, constructive thoughts intended to recondition the brain. You could repeat things like, for instance, regarding food addiction: "I am free of overeating. To recognize what to feed, I talk to my body. In reasonable quantities, I prefer to consume balanced foods. Sugary foods don't help me. Every day, I feel more confident."

Envisioning the Change—Once you have offered your constructive subconscious feedback, imagine how the better route would be pursued. See yourself live with a good connection to food. This enhances the concept and helps it to grab a root and maintain itself.

Who Can Give Hypnosis a Try?

Anyone who has difficulty committing to a balanced diet and workout regimen can, frankly, be a perfect choice because they do not appear to break their bad behaviors. It is a symbol of a subconscious issue to get caught in unhealthy patterns, including consuming the whole bag of Doritos instead of quitting when you're full.

Your brain is where your fears, behaviors, and addictions are housed. And it could be particularly powerful because hypnotherapy tackles the subconscious rather than just the awareness. In fact, a 1970 research review showed that hypnosis had a success rate of 93 percent, with fewer sessions required than both psychotherapy and behavioral therapy. It prompted researchers to conclude that hypnosis was the most powerful tool for modifying attitudes, thinking patterns, and actions.

Hypnotherapy also doesn't need to be used on its own. Hypnosis may often be seen as a supplement to various weight loss programs developed by physicians to manage common health problems, such as arthritis, obesity, diabetes, or cardiovascular disease.

Can Weight Control Occur with Hypnotherapy?

For individuals trying to reduce weight, hypnosis can be more successful than diet and exercise alone. The premise is that it is necessary to manipulate the subconscious to modify behaviors such as overeating. However, it is also up for discussion just how powerful it can be.

In individuals with sleep apnea, one earlier randomized study investigated the usage of hypnotherapy for losing weight. The research looked at two unique types of hypnotherapy for weight reduction and sleep apnea against simple diet guidance. In 3 months, all sixty individuals lost 2 to 3 percent of their body weight.

The hypnotherapy community had shed a further 8 pounds on average at the 18-month follow-up. The study found that although this extra loss was not as important as a cure for obesity, hypnotherapy required further study.

To live and function, we consume food. Although it's not necessarily because of whatever we eat. For every person, the cause resulting in emotional eating may most likely be different, but there can be certain similar emotions that induce emotional eating, i.e., consuming not to relieve hunger, but to attain respite for the moment from bad emotions. This is the unhealthy eating behavior that contributes to poor eating patterns and results in weight gain. Usual emotional eating causes are:

- Shame
- Poor self-esteem
- An impression of recurrent loss

- Loneliness

- Sorrow

- Grief

- Anger

- Fear

The real irony is: the aforementioned emotions cause emotional eating, but the shame and long-term mass gain arising from emotional eating will result in activating these emotions again! Emotional foodies instead opt for the refrigerator and eventually wind up feeling unhappier, instead of coping with anger and discussing the root of it.

The Stressful Emotional Eating Loop

We've learned that not only do human beings feed to relieve the need to eat. Emotional consumption is more about the usage of connections and signs. We are eager to allow one element to portray another, which typically fits us well in the creation of modern technology and highly advanced society. Yet we use comparisons and phrases very much in a derogatory way. We may also equate a particular pang of anger with a burst of hunger as we attribute this to emotional feeding. And it turns into a normal presumption in certain situations that feeding would fix the problem.

Then why turn it into a loop of emotional eating? And after we have eaten, the emotions of remorse that come in induce some of the similar emotions, and the loop starts again. This behavior is never deliberate; it just occurs. In a manner that is impossible to modify, we have programmed ourselves. Ever wonder why a dog turns nervous while in the kitchen and he senses the noise of tinkering? He connects the sound by making him a meal. This sort of connection is called Classical Conditioning.

Through the influence of hypnosis, hypnotherapy will help you transform long-standing behaviors.

Hypnotherapy will help you crack the cycle of emotional consumption by approaching the topic at the stage that's rooted in the unconscious mind. You can see some good things occurring over the process of the hypnotherapy:

- You become more comfortable, and thinking becomes easier.

- It will start to feel normal to hold the mental requirements and physical requirements apart and will thus arise naturally.

- You will search for more innovative ways to work the thoughts and work with them.

- Your appetite for nutritious food will grow, and your nutrition will change tremendously.

- In daily life, you will begin to turn more optimistic, more secure, and satisfied without a relentless cross to carry.

Chapter 15: Strategies for Maintaining a Healthy Relationship with Food

It happens when people start overeating or under food when they are overwhelmed with mixed emotions rather than eating in response to their inner cues. Strong emotions we experience can sometimes prevent us from listening to our physical feelings and thus preventing us from feeling hungry or full.

In such a scenario, food is used as a mechanism of coping, thus reducing the effect of the intense emotion temporarily. This habit is very addictive, and if not controlled, can lead to obesity, rapid weight gain, overeating, guilt, and shame. Stress-related eating disorders, if not handle, can make one vulnerable and not comfortable with their body.

This is where meditation plays a significant role because one will be able to handle their stress situation and, therefore, not use food as a coping mechanism.

Stress eating affects millions of people each year, and although not many will admit it can cause food addiction and unhealthy eating choices. As one eats, they believe eating relieve them of stress and often blame other people for their problems.

They do not see the need to eat healthy because their mind is preoccupied with so many things.

Dieting

Dieting only changes the food you eat for a while and limit your mindset.

Thus, Meditation will help you tap into your inner feelings and respond to your craving with the ability to control yourself.

Not being on a diet also makes you keep your focus because you will be keen on what you eat and how beneficial it is to your body. Meditation for weight loss changes the perception of the mind, which in turn triggers the inner self to respond to the choices and decisions made. Dieting is restrictive and specific on the meals you are to eat.

It challenges the mind to believe that restriction in terms of food is the only path to weight loss. Meditation, however, is a healthy way of letting the mind be free to choose what is best, learn from mistakes, and be able to focus on becoming better. It is possible to gain weight loss once one stops the diet process. It can offer both long-term and short-term weight-loss needs. However, the disadvantage is you must know the calories to take per serving. If you do not know, you may take less, and your body will be deprived of the needed nutrient.

Tackling Barriers to Weight Loss

There are so many barriers to weight loss from personal, to medical, to support system and emotional health. Meditation, if incorporated, will bring fruitful and healthy results. Dedication to overcome the challenges and to be focused on achieving your goals is significant. There are so many distractions, especially before you start your weight-loss routine.

It takes discipline and resilience to manage a weight loss program. We need to give weight loss the priority it deserves. Also, we need to realize the existence of the said barriers and their contribution toward our goal. The barriers will determine our successes and failures.

Set Realistic Goals

When you set goals, ensure that they are attainable, specific, and realistic. It is effortless to work on realistic goals and achieve them for better results. If the goals are unrealistic; however, the success rate will be low and you will be discouraged. For instance, when starting with meditation, you can start with as little as five minutes a day and gradually increase it daily until you reach the maximum time like sixty minutes.

The same applies to lose weight during the meditation process. You can start focusing on losing a few pounds each week and gradually increase until you reach your goal. As you set goals, however, realize that it is not your fault if they do not work out as you had planned, do your best and keep your focus.

Always Be Accountable

Once you have decided to commit to meditation for weight loss, don't shy away from sharing your plan with your support system and family. It is to ensure that the people you share with also reinforce the commitment and form part of the support system. That way, they will feel part of the program and give support whenever you need it. You can also use apps for reminders and timings; this way, you have a backup plan whenever you forget.

You can also use motivational bands whenever you achieve a milestone set. Being accountable makes you enjoy your successes, acknowledge your failure, and appreciate your support system.

People thrive when they feel responsible for something, especially for something beneficial to their well-being.

Modify Your Mindset

Your thinking needs to be modified in the sense that you be keen on the information you are telling yourself. Ensure that your mind is not filled with unproductive and negative thoughts, which will bring you down or discourage you. Do not be scared of challenging your thoughts and appreciate your body image.

Your mindset determines your thinking and in turn, creates a sense of appreciation or rejection. Our weight loss largely depends on our mindset, do you believe you can do it? If you think you have all it takes, then absolutely nothing will prevent or stop you.

Manage Stress Regularly

Having a stress management technique should be part of one's daily routine. You need to develop a healthy stress-relieving mechanism that can help you live a stress-free life. Understand that meditation is a stress reliever in its own right as it helps calm the mind and soothes the body.

It can be used to manage stress and its benefits fully utilized to live a more productive life. Be able to handle stress efficiently. Stress is not healthy for the mind.

If not handle, it can cause emotional problems and makes one irrational, moody, or violent. Be your own boss when managing your stress.

Be Educated About Weight Loss

As you embark on meditation for weight loss. Be educated about how it works; that way, weight loss will not be a struggle.

You will be able to handle failed attempts as well as appreciate the progress made.

You will be able to know what you have been doing wrong and decide on the best meditation exercise for you.

If you have misleading information, then your general progress may be inhibited

Weight loss need not be too expensive; neither does it require a costly gym membership or enrolment in a costly meditation class. There are various self-practice meditation exercises that you can comfortably do at home. Various meal plans and diets may work for others though they may not offer long-term solutions or lasting behavior changes. Have the right information that you need. Don't be misled by anyone posing that they are professionals in that field. Also, do not hesitate to do research online and compare notes. From there, you will be able to come back with something that works for you.

Surround Yourself with a Support System

There are people out there who may be ready and willing to help whenever you want to start or even after you have started.

The support system may include your family, colleagues, friends, or social networks. These groups of amazing people may encourage and support you to meet your long-term goal. After you include them in your plan, they will feel accepted, offer opinions, and check on your progress. Analyze how things are going, as well as encourage you to continue taking a little break when necessary.

Your support system should also include professionals in the field who will give sound advice and offer needed support and care.

Chapter 16: Mindfulness Exercise Techniques and Strategies

We are creatures of habits; by habits, we fall, and by habits, we rise. Why then not strive to develop those habits that will only lead to our uplift rather than our fall in life? To help achieve success in life, I have earlier shown you why you should avoid bad habits, and I have even some of the really ugly ones you need to avoid as well as their effects on your life. Here are some of the positive ones you should look to make a fixture of your routine.

Wake up Early

If those who have really achieved greatness in life slept for much of their time, they would not have become the people we know them to be today. While you may not have to stay awake in the night crunching lines of codes as Bill Gates did, you also do not have to spend more of your time in bed. Do not be slothful. Get enough good sleep; make a habit of a good sleep pattern, but that pattern should have you waking up early. The early hours of the morning are the most productive hours mentally. When you wake up early too, you get to plan your day out and set the ball rolling before half of the world knows it's a new day already. That you get to work or school early is just an added bonus.

Meditate

Meditation does not require you to subscribe to a belief system. It is just a system of deep reflection that can be used to achieve relaxation and peace of mind. You need your mind to be in the right state for the day's grind, and how better can you put your mental parts together than by meditation? There are many techniques out there, and you only need to get a book or read articles online about them. Meditation can be done in the morning, at work, or even after work in the evening. Meditation is one habit you will find in almost every great personality's life. It is that important.

Exercising

Health is wealth, they say, and you must seek to keep yourself in the best possible state of health. You can prevent sickness and stay in good shape physically and mentally by exercising regularly. Make a habit of exercising every morning (just twenty pushups or sit-ups can go a long way to set things right in the physical, biochemical factory we call the human body). If you make a habit of waking up early, you will have enough time to meditate and exercise. If you do not have enough time to exercise sufficiently in the mornings, you can always do it in the evening. You should just find a way to work it into your day.

Eating Healthy

You need to be careful with what you put into your body whether in the form of food, drink, and even drugs. Eating healthy is a must for good health. Food provides you with the right kind of nutrients you need for your work but only if you eat it in the right quantities and proportions. Eat

117

right and live right; that is the code. Together with exercise, eating right will help you stay fitter and fresher for longer to deliver success.

Read and Write

Reading makes a fine mind, writing an even better mind. These two acts help you grow intellectually. Through reading, you gain ideas that you never knew existed. It could even be an idea you know that is being shown in a new light. Reading increases your knowledgebase. But do you know what writing does? It gives clarity to your thoughts. It doesn't matter what you are writing; just put pen to paper every day. Put down your goals, aims, and plans; it gives them concrete form, and they take on a life of themselves when you put them down. You do not even need to be a superstar writer to put down the things in your mind for your own consumption. Write to yourself every day even if you do not intend to share with anyone. Reading and writing never harmed anyone. Rather, they could become your best tools for self-development.

Set Goals

After making a habit of all the mentioned activities, then, you need to learn to set goals. Too many people blunder through life with only a faint idea of what they want from it. Many are on a journey towards a vague destination. It's no wonder then that many end up arriving nowhere. You do not need to join this ill-fated trip. Rather, you are already in the ideal state of mind and physical health to be able to decide what direction you want to go in life. You should probably have read books on how to set goals and what goals to set. If you have not yet, I should tell you the first and most important rule of goal setting which is essentialism. This means you should not bite off more than you can chew. Determine the next right thing, and focus on it. Give it your all and move to the next thing on your plan. When you have achieved that thing, start the process all over for a new goal.

Perseverance

This is a very good habit that helps one sail through life smoothly. Life is never a bed of roses. The ups and downs that seem to pop each time one turns the corner seem insurmountable. However, with constant perseverance, you will be able to pass each difficult stage in life, mentally unscathed so that you have enough energy to move on in life with other endeavors. Perseverance is a mental habit rather than physical, but that does not render it any less important.

Positive Thinking

Nothing frustrates your efforts more than negativity. If you are not positive about your ability to get something done, you will do a shoddy job to validate your doubts. Negativity shows there is not enough enthusiasm to achieve something great. Make a habit of positive thinking, and you will stop seeing obstacles but already crossed hurdles. You can practice positive affirmations to boost your positive thinking.

Develop Money Management Skills

If you have a bad money-saving habit, you will never have enough for yourself. Perhaps a lesson can be learned in the story of Vanderbilt, the

119

great American philanthropist, and 11th-century millionaire. While working the sailing boats in America, Vanderbilt saved a lot until he got a better job on a ship and still saved a lot. In fact, he eventually bought that very ship and ended up owning a fleet. How did he achieve this? He made a habit of money management. He never spent impulsively and never fell for the constant invitation to acquire things just for the fun of it. Make a habit of monitoring your finances, and you will realize you are richer than you had earlier imagined.

Cultivate Social Skills

You cannot be an island unto yourself. You are human, and you exist in a human society. Whether you like it or not, you will have to relate with others. Why not do that in the best way it can be done? Cultivate good social skills online and offline. Learn to converse with people with pure and sincere intent. Smile at people, and they will smile back at you. Appear clean and neat always. Your appearance is your cover letter and calling card. Cultivate social grace and eliminate awkwardness. You will be thankful you did.

Chapter 17: Using Positive Affirmations to Lose Weight

What are Affirmations?

Most successful people in any walk of life have plenty to say about using positive affirmations and how the words contributed significantly toward the achievement of their goals. You cannot succeed and gain the long-term benefits of anything you want if you are constantly putting yourself down or have a mind that is constantly being weighed down by negativity. This negativity does not just have to be directed inward. This negativity can also be directed toward external sources like other people and certain circumstances. No matter the source of negativity, it breeds a negative mind.

Negative thoughts kill your zeal and enthusiasm in addition to sinking deep into your subconscious mind. They have the same power of guided meditation, whereby they need to make themselves a reality.

Therefore, if you are constantly thinking negative things about your body and your ability to gain your ideal weight then that is the reality that you will manifest. That is obviously not the reality that you want. As a result, you need to feed your subconscious positivity with positive thoughts and an inert belief that you will accomplish the things you set your mind to.

We are not born with this inert belief in ourselves, it is something that is developed. Ask any successful person that you know, from someone who has lost weight successfully or developed a successful career, and you will see that this person had to fight that internal fight to develop a positive mental environment. Of course, it is typically not an easy process but it is a doable process for the persistent, consistent, and tenacious.

Therefore, you can develop that belief, too. You can do this by feeding your subconscious with positivity and encouragement about yourself, your abilities, and your capabilities. Using positive affirmation allows you to have this power. It replaces your "I can't" trend of thinking with "I can" thinking, and that is infinitely powerful.

Positive affirmations are statements that you recite to yourself that describe a goal you have set for yourself but you say the statement in such a way that it comes across that this goal has already been completed. Just like guided meditation, these statements reprogram the subconscious but this power is not just limited to that part of the mind. Your words have the power to restructure your unconscious mind as well. Thus, they have the power to change how you think about yourself and the wider world. Fundamentally, saying positive affirmations changes your attitude, your behaviors, and, by extension, your life for the better.

The Benefits of Positive Affirmations

The benefits of positive affirmations are what make so that so many people swear by their usefulness and effectiveness. Reprogramming your mind by

122

your own power with an act as simple as repeating the same statements over and over again has the following advantages:

• Allows you to concentrate on your goals through a constant reminder.

• Creates the motivation to act on achieving your goals, especially when you start to see results from your actions.

• Develops new and improved beliefs about yourself and the wider world.

• Aids in changing negative self-talk into positive self-talk to foster a better mental and emotional environment.

• Allows you to put things in perspective.

• Allows you to be in a constant state of gratitude.

• Helps in boosting self-esteem and self-confidence.

• Aids in decreasing the symptoms associated with mental illnesses like depression and anxiety.

• Aids in improving sleep quality.

How Positive Affirmations Work

The use of positive affirmations is so powerful because they derive power from the Law of Attraction. The Law of Attraction sounds complicated but it is not. It is rather simple in fact. This law states that you and everyone else on this planet have the ability to attract the things that they want out of life by focusing on that desire then acting accordingly to gain that desire. This law does not discriminate. You can be whatever age, gender, religion, nationality, or race and it still works. The Law of Attraction is powered by the mind's ability to create the driving force that turns our thoughts into reality. The law is based on the premise that all our thoughts turn into reality at some point.

Therefore, if your focus is on doom and gloom, that is what you will manifest. If your mind is constantly occupied with thoughts of what a failure you are and how you will never lose the weight that you want to, then that will be your reality because you are manifesting your thoughts.

On the other hand, if you feed your mind positivity like what a winner you are and how you will lose the unwanted weight that you carry by your own virtue then that is what you will manifest.

Positive affirmations feed the mind positivity and uplift a person and their goals. The Law of Attraction dictates that these good thoughts will become reality eventually when you follow up those thoughts with massive action. Therefore, think that you are a winner then do the work to become a winner and the Law of Attraction will allow you to make that thought a reality. In the same way, the Law of Attraction says that if you think that you will shed the unwanted pounds then put in the work, those thoughts will become reality as well.

Guided Meditation and Affirmations

Guided meditation and affirmations make a great combo and we highly recommend that you use them in tandem. With guided meditation being a great way to impress positivity into the deeper levels of the mind, you can magnify that effect by using positive affirmations in your guided meditation scripts.

An easy way to incorporate the two techniques is to play your recorded positive affirmations when you are meditating. Ensure that the recordings capture the essence of what you are trying to impact upon yourself. Use your intonation and the inflection in your voice to say these affirmations like you truly mean them.

The great thing about hearing your own voice saying these affirmations while you meditate is that it makes the message more believable to all levels of your mind. Meditation makes the mind more receptive to receiving that message.

How to Prepare to Use Positive Affirmations for Weight Loss

There is a certain structure that positive affirmations must have for them to be effective enough to interrupt and then replace the negative thoughts and beliefs in your mind. The first thing you need to do is be frequent with the use of positive affirmations. You cannot use affirmation sometimes and hope to experience the benefits. Relate this to physically exercising and you will understand. You need to exercise regularly and consistently to gain the benefits of physical activity. Affirmations are an exercise regimen for your mind. You need to practice regularly and consistently to build that mental muscle. You need to flood your mind with positivity so that it washes away the negativity. This means using affirmations daily but not just once a day either.

There is no limit to the number of positive affirmations you can recite to yourself on a day-to-day basis. There is no special place you have to be or special time that you need to adhere to. All you have to do is be vigilant in monitoring the talk that goes on in your mind. Do not wait for a specific time to recite positive affirmations. If you notice your mind wandering into negative territory, instantly quell that flow by saying positive affirmations. That could be at your workplace when your colleagues or your boss gets on your nerves, when dealing with difficult family members or when you feel defeated by your workout regimen. There is no limit to how, when, or why you can use positive affirmations.

You can customize the words of your positive affirmation to provide inspiration and encouragement for whatever situation you need that inspiration or encouragement in. The reason that affirmations are so easily customizable is that they are based on you and your needs, not that of other people. You cannot control other people's feelings, thoughts, or actions but you can control your own. Positive affirmations give you that control.

Because positive affirmations are about you, they need to start with the word "I." Use the present tense when developing the statement. This gives your mind the visualization that this inspiration or encouragement is already a fact. Remember that the subconscious mind cannot tell the difference.

The statements need to be brief. They are only one sentence long. These statements need to also be positive. Always! You want to flood your mind and thus, affirm things that you want, not things that you do not want or negative things.

Positive affirmations need to also be specific. Do not beat around the bush when it comes to these statements. State exactly the desire that you would like to make a reality.

Finally, it is best to use words that express the emotions that you would like to achieve as well as verbs in your statements. They give your statements a dynamic form and so make this visualization a moving one in your mind—like a movie. We are all more stimulated by movies compared to a still picture.

How to Create Your Own Positive Affirmations

Creating positive affirmations is not complicated or hard. Below you will find an easy process for creating your own. Really, the hardest thing about positive affirmations is saying them with the enthusiasm necessary to convince your subconscious mind that they are true.

As you create your affirmations, write them down as much as possible. Writing has a way of making words more real to the mind. Also, set a schedule for regular positive affirmation recitals. We have said that positive affirmations do not need to be confined to a specific time (and we reinforce that statement), however, ensure that there are times especially dedicated to saturating your mind with positivity. Some of the times that most people see the best results when practicing affirmation recitation are in the morning as soon as they wake up, midway during the day to keep motivated, and just before going to bed. Any other time can be for reinforcement, as a reminder to stay strong, motivated, and encouraged during difficult times. You need to keep yourself accountable. Practice saying positive affirmation every day!

To create positive affirmations that are specific to you, the first thing you need to do is make a list of the things you think of as negative qualities about yourself. Listen to the negative self-talk that goes on in your mind and make a written note of them. When it comes to weight loss, list the things that you do not like about your body and the doubts you have about your capabilities when it comes to losing weight.

Next, change that negative into a positive. Examine the part of your body or the capability that you have these bad thoughts about but instead of being biased by negativity, examine these things objectively and search out the things you like. Sticking to your weight loss journey, your doubt might be you dread the physical exercise and thus, do not think you can keep it up. Objectively looking at this, you might realize that you can indeed do this because you are tenacious in other aspects of your life and there is no reason why you cannot apply that quality to working out.

Chapter 18: Tools for Thin Cognitive Behavior

Detecting brain hunger is the key to the rewiring process. We try to restore this ability when our anxiety level is in the stratosphere, or when we feel the pressure to participate in social ceremonies, or when we do not have access to masquerades where hunger exacerbates the problem. Mindfulness practices give us equality to physically recognize the body, more easily accept emotions, and protect ourselves from the unhealthy response to social pressures. If we're careful, instead of cutting off the overwhelming wiring depicted as desire (due to uncomfortable social circumstances, peer pressure, or inadequate emotions) and spending powerlessly, you can engage in alternative practices.

Meditation is most commonly referred to as a means of achieving mindfulness and thereby recognizing brain hunger. If the idea of meditation is actively provoking you (and this is understandable for today's modern-day women), try some form of active meditation (such as swimming).

Here are other helpful tips for achieving mindfulness without meditation:

For example, decide whether to return to mindfulness several times during a busy day, move slowly in your life, or be overly aware of your surroundings. An example of how you can become over conscious is to recognize something new every day as you walk through the park you want to walk.

The decisive factor is to be careful, and it just doesn't happen. By developing a Mindful Trigger, you can remind yourself to lead a conscious life. Remember, we have to be aware of the hunger of the brain, and we need to be aware of physical hunger. The success of repeating TCB steps accelerates and strengthens rewiring! These neural networks are restored when a food panic occurs and can calmly observe what is called brain hunger, and identify emotional needs that need to be addressed. This is an experience where you don't have to worry about it, and you don't overeat.

Mindfulness Aids

Following are some tips that will be helpful to obtain mindfulness:

- Laugh in Public—Laughing not only makes you feel better, but it also creates a positive energy exchange when you interact with someone.

- Name the mood—Running the same activity in different moods will produce different results. Note how mood affects biology?

- Reconnect with Your Body—Be aware of your body position and how it affects you. Is your body nervous or open and fluid?

- Return to yourself before being with someone—Breathe and return to yourself before interacting directly with someone by phone or email. When the phone rings, you need to be careful again. The caller makes you fresh, present, and available.

- Something old or new—become aware of something new when you are walking down a frequent path. There can be multiple things you can pay attention to, such as computer keystrokes, birds' chirping, the gentle roar of an airplane above you, or your footsteps, or many more.

- Pamper the child inside—it may be as easy as lying in the grass. It may seem silly at first, but don't let others decide your life. Feel the leaves, the breeze, and the sun on your skin. It always brings me back to that moment and gives me a mysterious, childlike feeling that lasts all day.

- Decide to go slow—it is nature that connects us again with the eternity of the moment. At each moment of this consciousness, we return to the title of the world phenomenon of Eckertall, "Power of Now." Torre wakes up his readers for a self-centered life as the creator of suffering and encourages them to live a painless life by living fully in the present. This book is highly recommended for anyone interested in learning the behavior of naturally lean women through the power of mindfulness.

Tools for Identifying Actual Needs and Responding to What Needs Attention

There are many causes for non-physical hunger: social situations (social hunger) that you think you need to eat to adapt, or if you feel socially uncomfortable and believe that overeating makes you feel good. If this can also be caused by an emotional imbalance (emotional hunger), we can't name it, deal with it, or develop it to calm ourselves. As your mindfulness develops, you will have more time to succumb to brain hunger as you better understand the causes of your brain cravings and take on the personal need for self-advocacy. Until the day overeating is history.

Part 2 of Step 3 is a feature that addresses all the needs of hunger. Once you have identified what needs your attention, you can develop skills that meet your needs rather than curb your needs. If we eat or eat too much, we continue the cycle of shame. By having the courage to name and address the underlying needs, we are strengthening a healthy neural network. So, most of it starts with emotions. Following are ways to recognize some of the emotions:

Blues

Low energy with no signs of physical hunger. In most cases, your dopamine levels are low. Moderately intense physical routine and/or meditation can increase dopamine levels to a considerable limit.

Boring

Remember that boredom is a form of self-rejection. It's important to work on one of your dream projects, the diary, the vision board, reconnect, and re-invest in one of your life's challenges. If you don't know what your interest is, promise to discover it from now on. There are thousands of resources and workbooks to help you with this search. Shift your energy towards this discovery process. This will take your attention and interest away from thoughts of food.

Disappointed

Express your disappointment clearly and loudly! Call friends, diary, scream! You do not need to stuff yourself with negative thoughts. You should share your insecurities and disappointments with the relevant people. Otherwise, they will lead to emotional imbalance and eventually to overeating.

Tired

If you overeat due to chronic sleep deprivation, investing in sleep hygiene best helps your ability to rewire your brain. Meditation is the number one recommendation for improving sleep quality as it calms the monkey. Start the "shutdown cycle" one hour before going to bed. Soothing music, low testosterone levels movies, soothing baths, sensual pajamas, dim light, no computer time, fewer excitement books, in short, a loss that increases the excitement.

Loneliness

If you are feeling lonely, you may call a friend. Go outside, meet someone. Do something good to someone, even strangers. Go to the hospice or children's crisis management center to help. The urge for food will subside, as the actual problem is mitigated.

Anger

If the problem is chronic, seek treatment from a specialist with anger expertise. If you are occasionally angry, make a loud voice, hit your bag, or walk while expressing anger. You may try to calm yourself by doing meditation or sleeping for some time.

Stress Accumulated

Work out or perform intense exercise. Scaling down to get the point of view, you have two options: indulge in worst-case thoughts (and increase stress and anxiety) or have the option to let go of your black and white thoughts. Observe meditation for the relief of stress.

Lost Control

Face your worst fear of what loss of control means to you in a general sense. Are you likely to concentrate on the worst scenario, the black and white way of thinking? Do you need control? What are you afraid of failing if you have no control?

If you don't know what you are doing, do a breathing exercise, reconnect to your body, and continue to ask quietly. "What do I feel?" "What is my energy level?" Important changes are exercise, meditation, using your favorite music, keeping a diary of your emotions, or taking a cold shower. It's something you can do immediately rather than unknowingly eat, and that's not a problem as long as you know it helps you pay attention to your real needs. Be prepared to repeat as many times as you need. If, for some

134

reason, you're limited and can't perform an alternate activity, imagine doing it carefully and in stages.

Chapter 19: How to Reduce Daily Calories Intake for Weight Loss

A calorie is a key estimating unit. For example, we use meters when communicating separation; "Usain Bolt went 100 meters in simply 9.5 seconds." There are two units in this expression. One is a meter (a range unit), and the other is "second" (a period unit). Essentially, calories are additional units of physical amount estimation.

Many assume that a calorie is the weight measure (since it is oftentimes connected with an individual's weight). That is not precise, however. A calorie is an energy unit (estimation). 1 calorie is proportional to the energy expected to build the temperature by 1 degree Celsius to 1 kilogram of water.

Two particular sorts of calories come in: small calories and huge calories. Huge calories are the word connected to sustenance items.

You've likely observed much stuff on parcels (chocolates, potato chips, and so forth.) with "calorie scores." Imagine the calorie score an incentive for a thing being "100 cal." this infers when you eat it, you will pick up about as much energy (even though the calorie worth expressed and the amount you advantage from it is never the equivalent).

All that we eat has a particular calorie count; it is the proportion of the energy we eat in the substance bonds.

These are mostly things we eat: starches, proteins, and fats. Sugars: 4. Calories: 2. Protein: 3 calories. Fat: 9 calories.

Are My Calories Awful?

That is fundamentally equivalent to mentioning, "Is energy awful for me?" Every single activity the body completes needs energy. Everything takes energy to stand, walk, run, sit, and even eat. In case you're doing any of these tasks, it suggests you're utilizing energy, which mostly infers you're "consuming" calories, explicitly the calories that entered your body when you were eating some nourishment.

To sum things up for you, NO... calories are not terrible.

Equalization is the way to finding harmony between what number of calories you devour and what number of calories you consume or use. If you eat fewer calories and spend more, you will become dainty, while on the opposite side, on the off chance that you gobble up heaps of calories, however, you are a habitually lazy person, and you will in the long run become stout at last.

Each movement we do throughout a day will bring about certain calories being spent. Here is a little rundown of the absolute most much of the time performed exercises, just as the number of calories consumed while doing them.

Step by Step Instructions to Count Calories

You have to expend fewer calories than you consume to get thinner.

This clamor is simple in principle. Calorie checking is one approach to address this issue and is much of the time used to get more fit. Hearing that calories don't make a difference is very common, and counting calories is an exercise in futility. Nonetheless, calories counting with regards to your weight; this is a reality that, in science, analyses called overloading studies has demonstrated on numerous occasions.

These examinations request that people deliberately indulge and after that, survey the impact on their weight and wellbeing. All overloading investigations have found that people are putting on weight when they devour a bigger number of calories than what they consume.

This simple reality infers that calorie checking and limiting your utilization can be proficient in averting weight put on or weight reduction as long as you can stick to it. One examination found that health improvement plans, including calorie counting, brought about a normal weight reduction of around 7 lbs. (3.3 kg) more than those that didn't.

Primary concern: You put on weight by eating a larger number of calories than you consume. Calorie counting can help you expend fewer calories and get more fit.

How to Reduce Your Caloric Intake for Weight Loss

Bit sizes have risen, and a solitary dinner may give twofold or triple what the normal individual needs in a sitting at certain cafés. "Segment mutilation" is the term used to depict enormous parts of sustenance as the standard. It might bring about weight put on and weight reduction. In general, people don't evaluate the amount they spend. Counting calories can help you battle indulging by giving you more grounded information about the amount you expend.

In any case, you have to record portions of sustenance appropriately for it to work. Here are a couple of well-known strategies for estimating segment sizes:

Scales: Weighing your sustenance is the most exact approach to decide the amount you eat. This might be tedious, in any case, and isn't constantly down to earth.

Estimating Cups: Standard estimations of amount are, to some degree, quicker and less complex to use than a scale, yet can some of the time be tedious and unbalanced.

Examinations: It's quick and easy to utilize correlations with well-known items, especially in case you're away from home. It's considerably less exact, however.

Contrasted with family unit items, here are some mainstream serving sizes that can help you gauge your serving sizes:

- 1 serving of rice or pasta (1/2 a cup): a PC mouse or adjusted bunch.
- 1 Meat serving (3 oz.): a card deck.
- 1 Cheese serving (1.5 oz.): a lipstick or thumb size.
- 1 Fresh organic product serving (1/2 cup): a tennis ball.

- 1 Green verdant vegetable serving (1 cup): baseball.
- 1 Vegetable serving (1/2 cup): a mouse PC.
- 1 Olive oil teaspoon: 1 fingertip.
- 2 Peanut margarine tablespoons: a ping pong ball.

Calorie counting, notwithstanding when gauging and estimating partitions, isn't a careful science.

In any case, your estimations shouldn't be thoroughly spot-on. Simply guarantee that your utilization is recorded as effectively as would be prudent. You ought to be mindful to record high-fat as well as sugar things, for example, pizza, dessert, and oils. Under-recording these meals can make an enormous qualification between your genuine and recorded utilization. You can endeavor to utilize scales toward the beginning to give you a superior idea of what a segment resembles to upgrade your evaluations. This should help you to be increasingly exact, even after you quit utilizing them.

More Tips to Assist in Caloric Control

Here are 5 more calorie counting tips:

- Get prepared: get a calorie counting application or web device before you start, choose how to evaluate or gauge parcels, and make a feast plan.

- Read nourishment marks: Food names contain numerous accommodating calorie counting information. Check the recommended segment size on the bundle.

- Remove the allurement: dispose of your home's low-quality nourishment. This will help you select more advantageous bites and make hitting your objectives easier.

- Aim for moderate, steady loss of weight: don't cut too little calories. Even though you will get in shape all the more rapidly, you may feel terrible and be less inclined to adhere to your arrangement.

- Fuel your activity: Diet and exercise are the best health improvement plans. Ensure you devour enough to rehearse your energy.

Effective Methods for Blasting Calories

To impact calories requires participating in exercises that urge the body to utilize energy. Aside from checking the calories and guaranteeing you eat the required sum, consuming them is similarly basic for weight reduction. Here, we examine a couple of techniques that can enable you to impact your calories all the more viably.:

1. Indoor cycling: McCall states that around 952 calories for each hour ought to be at 200 watts or higher. On the off chance that the stationary bicycle doesn't show watts: "This infers you're doing it when your indoor cycling instructor educates you to switch the opposition up!" he proposes.

2. Skiing: around 850 calories for every hour depends on your skiing knowledge. Slow, light exertion won't consume nearly the same number of calories as a lively, fiery exertion is going to consume. To challenge yourself and to consume energy? Attempt to ski tough.

3. Rowing: Approximately 816 calories for every hour. The benchmark here is 200 watts; McCall claims it ought to be at a "fiery endeavor." Many paddling machines list the showcase watts. Reward: Rowing is additionally a stunning back exercise.

4. Jumping rope: About 802 calories for each hour. This ought to be at a moderate pace—around 100 skips for each moment—says McCall. Attempt to begin with this bounce rope interim exercise.

5. Kickboxing: Approximately 700 calories for every hour. Also, in this class are different sorts of hand-to-hand fighting, for example, Muay Thai. With regards to standard boxing, when you are genuine in the ring (a.k.a. battling another individual), the biggest calorie consumption develops. Be that as it may, many boxing courses additionally incorporate cardio activities, for example, hikers and burpees, so your pulse will, in the long, run increment more than you would anticipate. What's more, hello, before you can get into the ring, you need to start someplace, isn't that so?

142

6. Swimming: Approximately 680 calories for each hour. Freestyle works, however as McCall says, you should go for a vivacious 75 yards for each moment. For an easygoing swimmer, this is somewhat forceful. (Butterfly stroke is significantly progressively productive if you extravagant it).

7. Outdoor bicycling: Approximately 680 calories for each hour biking at a fast, lively pace will raise your pulse, regardless of whether you are outside or inside. Add to some rocky landscape and mountains and gets significantly more calorie consuming.

The volume of calories devoured is straightforwardly proportionate to the measure of sustenance, just like the kind of nourishment an individual expends. The best way to lessen calories is by being cautious about what you devour and captivating in dynamic physical exercises to consume an overabundance of calories in your body.

Chapter 20: Creating Eating Plans for Success

Seek advice from a healthcare professional or registered dietitian before actually starting a new eating plan.

Low-Calorie Diets: Reducing your daily calories by less than 1400 calories per day would be detrimental because your body adapts to a semi-hungry state and is looking for alternative energy sources. Your body eventually burns muscle tissue, in addition to fat burning. But since your heart is a muscle it will be seriously damaged by times of starvation and tamper with its regular beats. Low-calorie foods do not satisfy the dietary requirements of the body and the body can't function properly lacking nutrition.

Appetite Suppressant Medicines and Other Diet Pills: "Wonder" items that irreversibly promote weight loss don't really prevail. Goods that guarantee instant or unobtrusive loss of weight would not work long term. Satiety suppressants, which often contain a psychoactive drug such as caffeine, are associated with health risks such as morning sickness, nasal dryness, agitation, anxiety, lightheadedness, sleeplessness, and higher blood pressure pres.

Fad Diets: Most fad diets promote consuming a lot of one form of food instead of a range of foods, which may be very harmful. Such forms of diets are also designed to manipulate consumers into wasting more on

144

unhealthy and even unproven goods. The best approach to consume requires balanced meals, so you can receive all the nutrition the body needs.

Liquid Diets: liquid dietary products or shakes that contain fewer than 1000 calories a day could be used under very strict professional monitoring. Such foods may be unhealthy and are not nutrient effective due to excessive amounts of sugar. There is also a very poor fiber content that induces blood sugar spikes and drops. Moreover, liquid diets do not reduce appetite, leading to the over-consumption of certain foods.

What's the Best Diet Approach for Healthy Weight Loss?

Pick up every diet book and it would falsely claim to contain all the keys to easily shed all the pounds you would like—and keep it all off. Many say that the trick is to consume less and workout more, some that fat-free is the only way to get there, and some recommend leaving out carbohydrates.

The irony is that there is no "one size fits all" approach for successful safe weight reduction. What works with one individual does not work for another because our bodies adapt differently to specific diets, based on biology and other health considerations. It is possible that choosing the best weight loss strategy for you would take time and include persistence, determination, and also some exploration with multiple diets.

Although some people react well to calorie counting or similar restrictive techniques, others react favorably to getting more liberty in organizing their weight-loss strategies. Simply avoiding fried foods or cutting back on processed carbohydrates could even set them up to succeed. So, don't be too downhearted if a regimen that worked for someone else doesn't work for you.

Remember: although there's no obvious answer to lose weight, there are still plenty of measures that can be taken to establish a healthful attitude towards food, reduce binge eating emotional triggers and sustain a healthy weight.

Keeping the Weight Off

You might have noticed the commonly cited figures that 95 percent of people trying to lose weight on a diet can recover it within a matter of years—or even months. Although there are not any concrete data to confirm this argument, it's clear that many weight-loss programs struggle in the long term. Maybe it's probably because overly stringent diets are really challenging to manage over time.

The (NWCR) National Weight Control Registry in the United States, since it was founded in 1994, has monitored over 10,000 people that have gained considerable quantities of weight and held it off over lengthy periods. The research showed that participants who have been effective in retaining their weight loss follow similar approaches.

- Stay fit and active. Prosperous dieters in the NWCR study exercise typically going to walk for around 60 min.

- Keep a food log. Recording your daily intake helps to keep you responsible and driven.

- Consume breakfast every day. It's most often cereal and fruit in the research. Consuming breakfast increases the appetite warding off cravings later that same day.
- Have more fiber than the standard American diet and less fat.
- Check your scale regularly. Trying to weigh yourself weekly may help you spot any slight weight gains, allowing you to take appropriate corrective actions even before a problem occurs.
- Watch less TV. Minimizing the hours spent seated in front of the television will be a vital aspect of having a healthier lifestyle and weight gain avoidance.

Hindrances in Weight Loss
Relying Too Much on Water

Drinking water is fantastic for the body. Although it is also claimed that consuming additional water then you'll need to ward off thirst is a magical weight losing trick—specifically consuming 6 to 8 glasses every day or more. Nevertheless, there is little confirmation that this will be effective. This turned out that drinking water, whether warm or room temperature, just expends a small number of calories. So focusing on this plan will not get you far from shedding pounds. On the other hand, people occasionally eat when they are really thirsty. And it is not a poor thing to quench the thirst before having a bite. It's always effective to approach for a drink of water than just a sugary drink, Pepsi or spice latte—any calorie drink can influence your quality of life, so there's no reason to think about it with water.

Sleeping Too Little—or Too Much

People put on some weight occasionally, for unexpected causes. One in four Americans isn't having enough time. And it could be that the shortage of sleep contributes to the obesity problem. Dozens of scientific studies have explored a link between obesity and sleep in infancy and several have identified a linkage. It is not clear if obesity makes it more difficult to have enough sleep or sleep which induces obesity. Many reports also aimed at people who are overweight. Such findings also indicate a correlation between increasing weight and getting more than 9 hours of sleep or below five hours. This could be due to hormone levels. Sleep cycles influence hormones linked to hunger and energy intake-burning-leptin and ghrelin. Besides that, individuals who sleep less generally feel fatigued and far less able to do workouts. Difficulty losing weight you might like to focus on sleep quality.

Relying on Restaurant Meals

Whether you have a full life or simply aren't a lover of home cooking, you place your body at the hands of the restaurants you buy from. Also, dishes marketed as "sweet" can contain more calories than you've been shopping from so several restaurants, especially smaller ones, don't mention their nutritional statistics so you can see what you're really consuming. There's even evidence that people who eat restaurant lunches outweigh those who prepare lunch at home by an average of five pounds.

Too Many Tiny Meals

You might have got to hear that trying to eat lots of small meal options all day long helps keep you fuller for longer without any excess calories. Yet to confirm this, there is barely any statistical evidence. Not only are tiny, daily meals stressful for preparing, but they may potentially end up backfiring, forcing you to consume more, and then once you start feeding, it may be hard to quit. If that is how you want to fuel your body, go for it. But it doesn't matter if your restricted-calorie diet is ingested all day long, or just three or four times a day. The most crucial part is having to eat a healthy diet with the proper calorie count.

Taking a Seat—All Day Long

Will that sound familiar to you? You are riding in the car to work, and going to a workplace where you are working for much of the day. You're worn out when you get home, and just want to—can you guess? Only sit down, maybe watch some television. All that sitting means your body doesn't move as much as it should for the best outcomes for your health. Studies have shown that those who spend more time sitting are more likely to weigh. But some studies say weighing more will lead people to sit more frequently. It's a complex process that affects the other, but here's something well known: while you're seated, you're not driving, doing housework, or standing up and running around a ton. All this energy that should be used eating up a few more calories by exercise, just through having a rest, health is sapped. And it can only benefit to take out more room each day to pass.

Overdoing Alcohol

Alcoholic beverages can expand your middle section more than you know. A beer, or two a day is popular among many Americans. But it sure does add up. Anyone that consumes two shots of vodka a day per week contributes about 1,400 calories to their diet—that's most calories in a day! And add still more wine and beer. Two bottles of wine a week contribute about 1,600 calories to the weekly count, and about 2,100 beers a day. So if you're willing to get serious about weight loss consider putting down the mug of beer for a while.

Rewarding Exercise with Food

Some people think that they can justify the extra help of pasta at dinner by working out. That may not however be the case. When we work out, we tend to overestimate the calories that we burn and technology doesn't help. Researchers find in one analysis that the typical aerobic unit overestimates on typical calories burnt by 19 percent. In that research, elliptical machines were the worst offenders, an average of 42 percent overestimating. That adds up to over a year's work out! Fitness bands have shown identical issues.

Turning to Snacks When You're Stressed Out

Have you ever learned of emotional eating? Eating can become an effort to fill an emotional vacancy within your life when you're stressed out. Sometimes this includes excessive snacking on high-calorie products, piling on pounds. One study had hair locks investigated for the cortisol stress hormone. For candidates who showed signs of long-term stress, they found a significant relationship between waist size and high body-mass index (BMI). None of this has a bright side to it. You can ease stress without having your wardrobe stretched out. Exercising can be the best way to both burn stress and lose weight. And relaxing techniques such as meditation, yoga, deep breathing, and massage can bring peace to your life—no calories needed.

Chapter 21: Mini Habits

Besides the meditation, your diet, and exercise routine, there are other smaller habits that you can use to discover the success needed to get in shape and keep it off. Here are some additional healthy habits that you can start actualizing in your life:

• Eat smaller bites

• Chew your food slower

• Don't clutch your utensils.

• Set aside an ideal opportunity for meal preparing

• Focus just on eating

• Stop purchasing unhealthy foods.

Attempt to remember these as you're going through your daily life. We will plunge further into them in this next meditation. By focusing your meditations on these, you'll see that it is easier to recall them. Doing these basic things can lead to some great outcomes.

Meditation for Healthier Habits

We will focus this meditation on shaping healthier habits. Tune in to this or repeat the content in your own voice and use that to help manage you through the meditation. Locate a comfortable position and start when you are ready. Let these thoughts course through your mind naturally, as if you

152

were saying them. I can feel each breath that enters and leaves my body. My breath comes in through my nose naturally. I don't have to consider it, and my body will breathe all alone. This is a habit that I created before I even left my mother's belly. I breathe faster when I am apprehensive. I breathe faster when I am energized. My breathing will slow as I become relaxed. At the point when I am falling asleep, I can feel my breathing going staggeringly moderate. My breathing will regulate itself. This is a habit that I have, and it reminds me I am human. When my breathing is happening in the winter, I can see it leave my body and make the air white. At the point when I am breathing on a hot sunny day, I can once in a while feel my warm breath on my body, making me feel significantly hotter. As I am breathing now, I see this theme. I perceive that habits are patterns that can come as naturally to me as breathing. Without considering it, there are a few habits that I take part in daily.

In the past, I have taken part in habits that were not healthy, and that is OK. I wasn't always aware of the unhealthy habits that I had shaped. Some things took somewhat longer to realize and it wasn't something I could always recognize all alone either. I can now perceive the unhealthy things that I have done in the past. These unhealthy habits included things like picking a diet I knew wasn't healthy for my body or choosing not to practice, although I realized I expected to get my body going. I won't rebuff myself because of these unhealthy habits. I am at peace with the decisions I used to make for my body. I will focus just on shaping healthy habits for me. I have to emphasize doing things that will better my body, mind, and soul later on. There is no better ideal opportunity to shape a healthy habit, then, I realize I have to remember it for my lifestyle. The better I can get at perceiving and adding healthy habits, the easier it will be to change my life. I am aware of the things I have to improve, and it is significantly easier to identify what I shouldn't do. I will always search for new healthy habits to remember for my life. I will recall that I have to keep investigating myself and guarantee that I am making the correct choices for the right reasons. There is nothing wrong with framing habits. Now I have to focus on framing healthier ones that will help me for a more drawn out timeframe. Habits will take time to shape. I won't have the option to frame all the habits I want for the time being. I will make sure I attempt every day to accomplish something healthy. From that point, I will locate the most natural habits to utilize, and the ones I have to alter to fit into my life more readily. I can shape healthy habits, as long as I commit myself to make healthy decisions every day. Some healthy habits will shape all alone. This is natural. Easy habits for certain individuals may be even more challenging for me, and that is OK. I will go at my pace, and the principal thing that matters is that I will be committed to adding these healthy habits. The more I focus on framing habits, the easier it will be to follow through with them. Habits will take as much time as it needs to form. It is OK to fall back into old habits; I have to have the solidarity to pull me back out. I will prepare for times when I may fall back into these habits, so I don't let it cause me disappointment. If I anticipate flawlessness all through my habit-framing process, I will just set myself up to feel defeated. Instead, I will prepare with encouraging affirmations and positive intuition, to help me through the occasions when I want to give up. Now is the best opportunity for me to enter the current world from this meditation, and to get focused on adding healthier habits to my life. I am going to put my mind towards guaranteeing that I include meditation as one of my habits, as this will improve my health. I start to leave this state of mind and come back to a superior, healthier place, situated on making healthy decisions. I can feel my breathing in a cadenced pattern that assists with relaxing my mind, body, and soul. I breathe in again, recollecting how it resembles a pattern, a mood, a habit. I feel the breath leave my body, exhaling the bad habits, inhaling the good. As I exhale the bad habits, I continue recalling how I can start these great habits as soon as my breathing has regulated. The time has come to be either focused or drift asleep at this point. As I count down from ten again, I will be out of this meditative state and back into the world that will assist me with forming healthy habits successfully. Ten, nine, eight, seven, six, five, four, three, two, one.

Chapter 22: Stop Procrastination

Probably the other bad habit everyone seems to have in life is procrastination. Some people may think waiting until the last minute is the key to success, but in reality, it is a double-edged sword that will kill you if you don't take care of it right. Sometimes you might work better under pressure, but procrastinating until the night before to do something and then staying up all night thinking about it can haunt you. You'll end up feeling worse than you've ever felt before. Procrastination comes to haunt you if you keep it around, and it's one of the worst habits out there. It will not only affect you but also the people around you. People rely on you, and if you're waiting on things until the last minute, you won't be able to be trusted. People will just think you're going to screw things up and keep everyone stressed. Plus, it's unnecessary stress, which is something that people don't need in this day and age. From work projects to school projects, to even just doing daily things, procrastination can affect anyone in all areas.

Procrastination might seem like one of those things that are unavoidable. After all, since everyone procrastinates, it's okay for you to do it. The thing is, it's not advisable to procrastinate on everything. Procrastinating on things will only cause more trouble than it's worth, and just because you're able to be successful with it once, doesn't mean it's going to work in your favor later on. You'll get addicted to doing things like this, and it will take your laziness to a whole new level until

156

you're able to face it. Which is usually when the deadline is right around the corner. You don't need that stuff in your life, and you can beat procrastination.

Look at the way you act when you procrastinate. Most people think that they work best under pressure, but in reality, getting things done actually makes a person feel better. Plus, you'll be able to look over the job and see if there are any mistakes, and you'll be able to polish it. You'll be able to improve your skills and abilities, and instead of turning in something that is made in a rush, you'll be able to turn in something perfect that people will enjoy.

Some people think that procrastination is the best thing ever. They say that it gets you motivated, but in reality, it stresses you out and causes you to make hasty decisions without thinking. You'll be putting extra stress on yourself, which isn't bad if it weren't for the fact that you probably have about ten other things to think about. The stress plus the procrastination causes you to switch moods and become emotional over everything. People become crazy when they're under stress, and not in a good way either. Procrastination can also bring out the worst in people, and some might be turned off from talking to you until you're done with screaming to the high heavens at them because you didn't' finish your project on time. Think about the stress that procrastination causes you. If you got it done early, you wouldn't have to worry about spending all that time worrying and you'll be able to spend more time feeling happy and accomplished.

Procrastination can also affect your sleep and nutrition. That's another thing that you have to think about and analyze. Procrastination usually causes people to stay up all night, leaving them dead tired the next day. The tiredness causes them to be less rational and will make them think that illogical things are sensible. They'll think that something they put in the project is correct when in reality they're dead wrong. It's not something that can help you. Instead, it will drain your energy and cause you to be an energy-starved mess until the project is over. It's the same in the food aspect of things. Food and nutrition are important for you to stay focused. When people procrastinate, they might go almost an entire day without eating anything, and most of the time they're spending their time living off of energy drinks and junk food. That will cause your body to become unhealthy, and the health problems will come to bite you over time. Food and nutrition is something that you need to think about, and if you're having issues with anything regarding nutrition and sleep, you should stop procrastinating before it gets worse.

A final bad thing about procrastinating is that it doesn't always work. Most of the time, the person gets lucky if the boss or teacher likes it, or if they get what they need to be completed on time. One might think that procrastinating is the way to success, but that's far from the truth. In fact, most of the time, procrastinating will make you perform worse because you're working so fast to get this whole thing done that you need to worry about that instead of making sure that you're at the top of your game. It's a shame, but most people don't realize that and think the lie of "procrastination is the key to success" is a truth. It's not, and you'll only feel miserable in the end if you do that. Most of the time it stops being as effective once you realize just how different your potential is when you do things early and take your time with it.

Now that you know what can come out of being a procrastinator and just how ugly it can be, it's time to look at the ways to change it. Yes, you can change your procrastination in some simple steps, and you'll soon see that it's not as hard as you may think. Most people think the idea of changing your behavior is the hardest thing in the world to do. In reality, it's not and people need to realize that. You can change the way you act and your habit of procrastination with these simple steps, and you'll see after a while that things are better if you do them when you first get them instead of trying to finish everything at the last minute like most people.

Now, the first thing to do after you recognize the problems of procrastination is to look at how you can stay on top of things. It might be something as small as a little reminder or as big as making a calendar of events. Take a look at how you can personally stay on top of your game and make sure you don't miss a thing. It's advisable to get a calendar and start filling it out. People need to look at things over a general period of time. You can't just think only looking at the next day is the best thing. You need to look into the future and plan for the future, for if you don't you'll only create issues later on.

Some might not like the calendar method, and if they don't, they can just write down what they need to get done in life. This can be a list of a few things or one with hundreds of things. Look at everything that you need to get done, and then divide it into smaller and smaller increments. This is similar to the way you manage your time, but this is related to just the project or the set of things you need to get done. Just put them all in and set up a list of them. Then, you can check off everything that you do to keep on top of your game.

With the calendar method, put the dates down for when things need to be turned in. It might be nice to do just that, but you're going to end up procrastinating if you just leave things at that. That's the lazy way to do things. In this instance what you need to do is schedule out each day what you need to get done to make that target for the day so that you can reach your goal with ample time to spare. Some days might be easier than others, but if it is easy one day, look over the work that you have done on the action and make sure everything is okay. You want to make sure that everything is in order and monitored each day. You don't want to put everything on one day. That's the way you've been doing it before, and that only leads you down a path you don't' want to take. Instead, stretch it out over some time. You'll soon see that it's not as bad as you think it is either.

If you're trying to procrastinate because you think the project is too big, think of the way things will be if you leave it like that for that long. You'll think that it's okay to leave it like that for three weeks because it's a giant project, but it's only going to look bigger as time goes on. Instead of worrying about things like that for an extended time, just do it now and chip away at it. You'll have way less of a headache if you do. Plus, if you spread it out for a couple of weeks, you'll see that it's not that bad. That will allow you to be in control of it and not be affected by it.

Once you have everything laid out, it's time to be motivated about it. The motivation can be as small as feeling happy that you got the thing done, or it can be the happiness of not having to worry about it. You're probably going to have to push yourself at first. Most people who want to stop procrastinating after being a procrastinator for so long have a hard time with this. But, if you just remember that there is something good at the end of it, you'll see that it's worth the fight. You need to have the motivation so it'll be the best thing for you to have when it comes to dealing with the stresses of finishing the project.

Chapter 23: Practical Steps to Stop Emotional Eating Disorder

Consider keeping a binge-eating diary. You don't need much for this; a standard planner will do (depending on how often you binge eat, really). In it track what caused you to binge eat. You'll be surprised with how quickly you'll start noticing patterns that you might otherwise have been completely unaware of. Often just a week is enough. Armed with this knowledge you'll then have a much better picture of what it is that is setting you off.

Manage Stress

As you'll notice from your diary, your cues are often stressed or anxiety-related. The first thing you, therefore, need to do is eliminate as many of these stress factors. Your work is setting off binge eating? Don't take your work home with you. Talk with the in-house psychologist about what stress management suggestions they might have. And if all that doesn't work, consider finding a new job.

Perhaps it's a social situation with a loved one? If you believe they're open for a conversation about such topics suggest, without accusation, that you find interacting with them stressful and that this is affecting you negatively. If you don't think they're capable of this kind of conversation without judging you or causing you discomfort then perhaps consider taking some time away.

162

Where you can't eliminate stress, manage it instead. There are stress-management strategies that can help. These include meditation, exercise as well as fun, and relaxation. These are all healthy ways to reduce the effects of stress in your life and if you can manage to replace your binge eating with any or all of these activities that might already help.

Plan on Eating Three Meals a Day

Don't skip breakfast. This is something that quite a lot of binge eaters do and it plays right into their binge eating. It has been shown that people that do not eat breakfast are more at risk of heart attacks and are more likely to be overweight than those who do eat breakfast. So, all those health benefits you were thinking you were getting, they aren't there.

How does avoiding breakfast do all these things? The reason is twofold. First off, by skipping breakfast you're continuing the fast from the previous evening onwards. Or, put more succinctly, you're starving yourself for longer. This causes all kinds of stress responses in your body, which aren't healthy and actually lead to calorie retention as your body slows down calorie consumption to help you cope. Then, when you do eat later on, because of your hunger it's going to be far harder to resist junk food cravings and eat healthily. Finally, it can lead to a disconnection between your stomach and your mind.

So, the long and the short of it is, eat breakfast! Try to take in at least some fruit and perhaps a bowl of cereal in the morning. From there try to expand your breakfast into something healthy that will keep you satisfied until lunch.

Also don't skip lunch or dinner. Plan to get three square meals a day that gives you the nutrition and the satisfaction that you need. That last part is important. If you're not enjoying the food you're eating, then there's a good chance you'll use that as an unconscious excuse to indulge (read binge eat) at some point along the line. This is not to say that you should eat burgers every day, but it does mean that you don't have to eat your boring vegetable salad every day either. Make certain that there are some aspects of what you're eating that you enjoy.

Enjoy Healthy Snacks

It's also a good idea to have healthy snacks on hand for when you have a craving for something. Again, this does not mean "boring." You're not trying to punish yourself. That will ultimately just trigger another episode of binge eating. Instead, look for something you like. There are quite a few snacks available on the market nowadays that are actually quite tasty without being loaded up with sugar, salt, or fat. This includes fruit but might also include nutritional bars and nuts. It depends on what you like really.

Establish Stable, Healthy Eating Patterns

Stability is your friend. For that reason, try to make arrangements so that you eat at regular times, preferably with other people as meal times are great occasions to socialize. If you don't have anybody to eat with, don't worry. That will change once you're back to a more normal and healthy ritual.

The first step towards that goal is to standardize your meal times so that your body once again gets used to more normal rhythms. This will allow your brain and your stomach to reconnect and thereby make you more aware of when you are hungry and when you're satiated. This will make it easier to stop when you need to. Also, don't eat in front of the TV. When you do so, you're more likely to overeat as it takes longer for you to become aware of signals from your stomach telling you that you've had enough.

Avoid Temptation

If you live with somebody else who occasionally likes to have junk food in the house, talk with them and ask them to help you overcome your problem. Yes, that does mean asking them not to keep junk food lying around where you can find it. It doesn't have to be permanent, just until you've got your binge eating under control.

In order to avoid temptation when you're in the supermarket or other places, don't go shopping when you're hungry. This is a very valuable piece of advice that won't just help your binge eating problems but will also help you avoid overspending, as everything always seems far more enticing when we haven't eaten. So, before you go to the supermarket or the mall, make sure you have a meal. This will make the entire experience far easier for you personally and your wallet as well.

Exercise

There is very little in this world that exercise isn't good for. It fights negative attitudes; helps you lose weight and generally makes you feel

165

better about your situation by flooding your system with endorphins and other happy chemicals. What's more, it will help you fight both boredom and stress, get to bed on time, and improve your energy levels. And though you might not believe it in the beginning when you're just getting started and your body is not used to it, many people find it quite enjoyable!

The trick is to exercise and not torture yourself. A lot of people, including trainers, seem to believe that the only way to gain is through pain. That is nonsense. The only thing that will cause is for you to hate exercising and feel resentful. That won't benefit anybody.

Instead, a much better strategy is to start slowly and then build up. In this way, you won't feel resentful for what you're doing and you'll have the enjoyment of seeing an improving line. Sure, this does mean that it will take a little longer before the effects of the exercise start to show, but on the flip side, it also means that the chance you'll keep going is much more significant.

If you weren't doing any kind of exercise, start by going walking or riding a bike. Initially, it doesn't have to be that far, as long as you've got a steady rate of improvement built-in. Today a mile, tomorrow a mile and a quarter. After that, think about joining in with a group. Here again, you mustn't go overboard and join the super hardcore do-or-die group, but something more at your level. Water aerobics, stretching exercises, or other forms that will push you but not break you are the best to start with.

If you are obese or overweight, initially you might not see much weight loss. Don't worry about that. You're still changing. It's just happening on the inside. You'll be transforming fat into muscle, for example. Only after that, the actual weight loss will start setting in. Don't get discouraged. Instead, look at what you can do, rather than how slim you are. Perhaps keep an exercise calendar in which you track what you did and how you feel. Then, consider you're at least straining yourself; you should see steady improvement.

Dealing with Boredom and Avoiding "No"

It isn't just in terms of food that you should avoid the "no" word, you should avoid it as a whole. So, don't just exclude binge eating from your life, find an alternative way to fill your time. So, take up a hobby. Better yet, continue a hobby that you used to have but had to let go of as a result of binge eating—something you really enjoyed and you feel you should be able to enjoy again. In other words, fill your time. Otherwise, boredom will set in, and then you'll spend your time trying (and failing) to not think about binge eating.

Get other people involved. Join a team or a class where other people come to depend on your presence. This way, even if you're having a down day, you'll be far more likely to go. Before you go you might not believe that you can actually enjoy yourself, but that will often change once you get there. In psychology, we call this the hot-cold empathy gap. It means that we can't imagine how something will feel unless we're feeling it. It's why temptation is so hard to resist and why we can't believe we can't resist it when we're not feeling it.

It's also why we can't imagine enjoying something outside of the house if we're sitting in it depressed and unhappy, but once we're outside of the house we find it quite easy to enjoy ourselves. And it is the reason why it's a good idea to take up activities where it isn't just our expectation of enjoyment that will get us to go, but also social commitments.

You could also consider getting a dog. These can offer you a great deal of companionship and also offer you opportunities to go for walks, which is obviously a great way to get exercise. Now, this goes without saying, but you must actually want a dog, as they do require a lot of attention and love. Don't get one if you're not sure about it, as otherwise, you'll feel bad about yourself and about not taking care of the dog!

If you are considering getting a dog, may I advise astray rather than a thoroughbred? Your local pound will have dogs that need homes or will be put down otherwise. Save yourself by saving a dog.

Chapter 24: Step by Step Guide to Stop Overeating

We need food to endure; however, when does require food arrives at a point where it brings indulging? When is it essential to take a look at yourself, make a stride back, and quit eating?

Each individual who has an unfortunate relationship with food see it likewise. It often fills in as a solace and security method that permits us to persuade ourselves that it is adequate to expend food carelessly and without deduction. Obviously, except if you are prepared in sustenance or value thinking about your prosperity, you most likely don't have a positive relationship with food.

Change Your Eating Habits

Suppose you've perceived the need to construct a superior relationship with food, and you might want to find more about hypnosis for weight loss and to kick your negative behavior patterns. In that case, you need to identify the underlying reason adding to your concern. Since eating introduces itself as a type of transitory pressure alleviation and diverts us from feeling feelings like pressure, pity, uneasiness and outrage, it's something we tend to incline toward at any rate eventually in our lives. Given that promoting organizations are specialists at giving defective society nourishments that may appear to be engaging or are canvassed into some degree "dietary-accommodating" content, we have embraced the

169

conviction that it is alright to expend artificial food or whatever advertising recommends to us. We have similarly instructed ourselves that expending unfortunate food goes about like a prize for whatever we're doing well.

Try Not to Punish Yourself

For example, revealing to yourself that you can eat anything you desire throughout the end of the week after five non-weekend days of clean eating is to count off-base. We ought not to be feeling like we are rebuffing ourselves by eating a whole, adjusted diet. It should turn out to be natural to us as we receive a sound lifestyle.

The initial step to utilizing hypnosis for weight loss effectively is identifying the reasons why you battle to accomplish whatever it is you need. When going through self-hypnosis, you should figure out how to address your food fixation and transform it into something valuable, for example, inspiration to not feel as powerless or wasteful as you do at your current weight or condition of wellbeing. Before you start with your meeting, you ought to recognize the motivation behind why your objective appears to be so far off, just as what it is that is keeping you away from accomplishing it.

What Will the Hypnotherapy Session Be Like?

During an expert hypnotherapy meeting, a specialist will, for the most part, ask you a rundown of inquiries identified with weight loss, including inquiries regarding your diet and exercise propensities. Since you are directing the treatment meeting all alone, you can just go over your day-by-day schedule and propensities. Once in a while, it assists with recording both your positive and negative propensities to see where you have to improve. You have to format the entirety of the data before you and spotlight on what it is you have to improve during your meeting. Recording your objectives will likewise assist you with building up a more clear image of where it is you'd prefer to go. Remember that self-hypnosis is completely up to you, so you need to submit and remain trained all through the 21 days.

This period is feasible for most people and sets a benchmark for yourself without making a responsibility that is too huge.

Since you need to rethink your food dependence, it's critical to speak the truth about unfortunate propensities with yourself, which could incorporate anything from pigging out, enthusiastic eating, indulging or deceiving yourself to accept that you need more food or most usually blamed, revealing to yourself that you'll begin a diet on Monday.

Providing essential facts about yourself and your propensities will allow you to find what you need to address and stand out.

The Importance of Setting Goals

Participating in hypnotherapy, you will have the option to improve your certainty through good proposals set out to cause you to feel engaged. Reevaluate your internal voice, which will remind you to keep a good and sound mentality, imagine yourself accomplishing your weight loss objectives, identify oblivious examples that prompted your present unfortunate lifestyle, just as dispose of any dread you may have in accomplishing your objectives.

You likely didn't realize that you could live in dread of accomplishing your objectives. It sounds absurd, yet changing yourself, or how you live could introduce itself as upsetting as well. Often individuals don't accomplish their objectives because they are dreadful of leaving their customary range of familiarity. Since we can't flourish or develop without being awkward in life, it's essential to defeat such dread feelings. Hypnosis will address your propensity designs and permit you to eliminate them from your psyche. It will permit you to grow new and feasible methods for dealing with stress. For instance, you can imagine yourself reacting to unpleasant cooperation or circumstance with hypnosis and pick how you might want to respond very steadily. You will likewise envision yourself eating well during the meeting to help you settle on better decisions and structure lasting dietary patterns.

Envision Success

To the individuals who don't battle with portion and needing control, think that it's easy to adhere to their standard eating method. Contrasted with somebody who is habitual and eats dependent on their sentiments, hypnosis is most likely the best technique for self-improvement. It works by controlling responses and propensities, which has clearly prompted your entanglements and unfortunate relationship with food. During the hypnosis meeting, you are prescribed to figure out how to dispatch your food desires and wipe out unfortunate propensities encompassing portion control. This causes you to envision yourself having a lot more advantageous relationship with food, which will set you up for progress.

With hypnosis, it appears senseless to simply zero in on genuinely getting in shape. There are so numerous different elements included that ascribes to what in particular causes weight gain that you can rectify. Getting in shape and accomplishing any wellbeing related objective is an excursion that will show you a way to carrying on with your best life.

The Most Effective Method to Eat the Right Amount of Food

To recover legitimate portion control and eat the perfect food measure at every supper, you have to zero in on eating the correct kinds of food. At exactly that point, you will have the option to keep up a reasonable diet. It's consistently useful to lead a little exploration before you start with hypnosis, particularly if you will likely figure out how to decrease your portion sizes and stick to it. Although you know the reasons why you should and that eating an excessive amount of food adds to the pointless store of fat that gets put away in your body, many individuals actually gorge notwithstanding. It's essential to advise yourself that you shouldn't be living to eat, but instead, eat to live. When you've built up this standard, you can control your portion sizes and, at last, get thinner.

If you practice hypnosis or are as of now following a diet, and you're not getting thinner, then you most likely need to assess your portion sizes. You likewise need to tune in to your body and realize whether the kind of food you're devouring is serving your body well. Conveying abundance weight

173

could be a consequence of gorging at suppers. Additionally, indulging every now and again is equivalent to eating an awful diet; it's bad for your general well-being or weight loss venture.

Digestion

Legitimate portion control alone won't cause you to lose all the weight; however, it will give you more energy, especially because continually being full places strain on our real cycles to work more enthusiastically. This incorporates your digestion, which, if not working proficiently, could make you clutch overabundance weight, to count stop your weight loss results, and cause you to feel awkward. Having frail digestion and insufficient processing could act as a genuine medical problem and incorporate problematic manifestations, for example, ongoing fatigue, weight gain, melancholy, cerebral pains, blockage, and sugar yearnings.

The expression "portion control," alludes to eating a satisfactory measure of food. The amount of what you devour, alongside the sort thereof, is required if your objective is weight loss. Often, individuals constrain themselves to complete the food on their plate out of amenability or because we can't perceive that we've had enough.

Chapter 25: How to Maintain Mindful Eating Habits in Your Life

Indeed, even with the best program and all the help on the planet, we as a whole have days when we could utilize some additional motivation. Here are a few things you can do to build your inspiration and assurance of your weight reduction achievement.

Set Achievable Goals

Something I can't pressure enough is the significance of making changes that you will have the option to stay with for an amazing remainder.

Start by defining little reachable objectives that aren't attached to a number on a scale. For example, rather than making it your objective to lose 10 kilos, why not intend to drink eight glasses of water each day. Or then again plan to take the stairs every morning on your approach to work. Another very accommodating objective is to tune in to your entrancing recordings, in any event, four times each week.

Whatever your objectives, ensure they are quite certain, unmistakable, and simple to achieve.

More activity is critical to wellbeing and when you are attempting to shed pounds it makes a difference like never before. Be that as it may, it is anything but difficult to get exhausted with the regular old exercise schedule for quite a while. Try not to stall out stuck!

175

Have a go at something new. Take a walk, take a yoga class, or investigate your neighborhood with a morning climb.

Exercise doesn't need to be done in a rec center, on a bit of gear, or with a teacher. You simply need to get going!

Prepare for the New You

Prepare for the new form of yourself that you are making. Wipeout any unfortunate nourishment from the cabinets. Dispose of old garments from the wardrobe. Modify your condition to suit the new life you are building.

Try not to Give in to Guilt

Nobody is immaculate and we all need a little chocolate sometimes. The main wrong thing with the infrequent guilty pleasure is the blame you feel a short time later. There is no point making yourself feel so awful about that one binge to spend that it thumps you to count off track and you wind up eating ten chocolates just to feel good. Normally flimsy individuals don't feel regretful when they have a periodic treat. They relish the experience and afterward get directly back to eating good foods. Blame isn't valuable—let it go!

Kevin's Story: Seeing the Hidden Price Tag for Unhealthy Food

Kevin was a foodie. He wanted to eat. He additionally adored biking and drinking wine. Be that as it may, those three things didn't appear to go together very well since he regularly drank excessively a lot of wine and didn't want to ride, and also, he had an additional 15 pounds he had been attempting to shed throughout the previous five years. The additional weight made riding with his companions harder and he hadn't had a ton of fun as of late for that very reason.

He came in for trance since he needed to curtail his drinking and gorging, get in shape, and become a superior cyclist.

Kevin's issue was not quite the same as Patty's: he could go for quite a long time without food, regularly working through lunch, and having very late meals. Yet, he likewise accepted an existence without great wine, cheddar, and the pastry wasn't one worth living. He really had an image in his mind of himself getting a charge out of wine, cheddar, and pastry with companions after a decent ride, and his bicycle was out of sight of this image. This was a picture he made that speaks to his optimal life and it fulfilled him to consider it. It likewise was a piece of what was making him over-enjoy because Kevin wasn't seeing the full picture—the genuine expense of what an overindulgence of high-caloric food and liquor was doing to his body. For Kevin, it wasn't as a lot of a constraining conviction as it was not seeing reality with regards to the decisions he was making.

Mesmerizing can assist us with distinguishing and be freed of restricting convictions on account of Patty and Jessie, however, it can likewise assist us with seeing things for how they really are. What's more, for example, when I say "see things" what I mean is that individuals are envisioning something in their brain—regardless of whether they're seeing it or simply thinking about it. Not every person really makes pictures in their mind.

I'll utilize "see" until further notice. For certain individuals, considering things to be what they really imply, as opposed to considering treats to be something that will satisfy them, they consider it to be something that fulfills them for 10 minutes, at that point liable and pitiful the remainder of the day. It implies seeing a glass of wine not as a pressure reliever, yet as a depressant that is really noxious to their body. A few customers will really change the image in their mind—they envision their preferred bag of treats with a scowling face on them, or an image of the genuine expense—them at their heaviest. Since that is an increasingly exact picture of what the treats will do. Imagine a scenario where makers were required to put outwardly of items what truly happened in the wake of consuming them. Okay, purchase a pack of chips with an image of overweight and despondent individual staring at the TV on the front. Shouldn't something be said about a piece of candy with an image of overweight and blame ridden individual outwardly? Also, shouldn't something be said about that pack of foods from the drive-through or take out—an image of you feeling worn out and drowsy?

Next time you buy an item, envision the bundling as having a picture of you 15 minutes after utilization. Perceive how that changes things for you. That is the truth in publicizing.

Hypnosis helped give Kevin the concentration and attention to comprehend what he was truly doing—on the scenario that he enjoyed the flavor of food and wine a lot, was a second or a third glass really vital? Is it accurate to say that it was even that great constantly glass? Genuine wine authorities let their wine out in the wake of tasting it. Shouldn't something be said about eating the whole bit of his preferred cheesecake—was that tenth nibble on a par with the first?

Kevin understood the genuine expense of his extreme drinking—it was constraining his profitability at work, and it was shielding him from being a superior cyclist. He understood if he genuinely cherished the flavor of wine, one glass would be sufficient. More than that, and he may have an alternate issue.

Portioning Your Food
1. Toss Out Your Scales

Do you think flimsy individuals bounce on the scales each morning? No, they don't. Fixating on the scales makes you a captive to them. At the point when you lose a pound or two, you may feel extraordinary, yet if you increase a little, at that point it can set you into a winding of implosion. The sentiments of disappointment that pursue can send you running for the closest bar of chocolate or another food comfort.

Also, restroom scales are not a precise method to screen your weight. Imagine a scenario where you are practicing more and picking up muscle. Or then again perhaps you need a decent solid discharge—well there goes a couple of additional pounds? Women, is it that time and your body is puffed up with liquid weight? Such a large number of components can impact that number on the scales.

So, it's a great opportunity to quit deciding your prosperity by what you gauge and start taking a gander at all the positive changes you are making in your life. Give the way you feel and the sound decisions you make a chance to be your new weight reduction indicator. Or on the other hand, essentially watch as your garments get looser and your body gets littler.

2. Tune in to Your Body

Pause for a minute or two to inquire as to whether you feel extremely eager. There are moments when we think we feel hungry, however just not many when we are really eager.

Frequently we feed our sentiments as a result of a bogus enthusiastic craving. Or on the other hand, perhaps we both feeling anxious for feeling hungry.

Genuine hunger is that slight chewing or void sensation in your stomach. Set aside an effort to tune in to your body, to truly tune in to your body's needs. Eat possibly to fulfill genuine craving and stop when your body has had enough. Pick food sources that make you feel fulfilled, supported, and light, and keep away from all foods that make you feel substantial, enlarged, and awkward. It's as straightforward as that!

3. Bite Your Food

Processing starts in your mouth and great assimilation is basic to changing the food you eat into the energy your body needs. At the point when you bite your food, it invigorates the discharge of stomach-related catalysts in your stomach and stomach-related tract. If you eat too rapidly, these proteins don't have the opportunity they have to process your food viably. At the point when you eat rapidly, you likewise swallow more air and ingest bigger parts of food which put a strain on your stomach related framework and can cause swelling and gas.

Additionally, the appetite hormone Leptin will keep on expanding as you eat, until your hunger has been satiated. Biting your food altogether and eating gradually gives your body time to perceive that it is full and permits leptin to communicate something specific from your stomach to your cerebrum to quit eating since you have had enough.

4. Eat Smaller Meals More Often

Eat no less than each 4-5 hours to give your body the fuel it needs to work effectively. This will help keep up your glucose levels and keep your digestion firing up. Plan with the goal that you have sound food close by consistently. Keep in mind that you need to eat when you begin to feel hungry, not after you become covetous. At the point when you experience over the top appetite, it is an indication of low glucose levels which will make longings for sugar and other bad food.

5. Make the Most of Your Food

Plunk down, slow down, unwind and make the most of your food. Making a loose and charming climate when you eat, urges you to bite bigger, eat all the more slowly, and makes it simpler to listen to your body. Likewise attempt to abstain from whatever occupies your concentration away from food, for example, sitting in front of the TV. Along these lines, you are bound to stay focused on the amount you are eating. The more cognizant you are of the point at which you are eating, the more you will tune in to the sign saying you have had enough.

Chapter 26: How to Avoid Getting Off Track

Telling a person to adopt the mentally strong traits is an excellent way to develop mental toughness, it may not always be enough. It's a bit like telling a person that to be healthy, you need to eat right, exercise, and get plenty of rest. Such advice is good and even correct. However, it lacks a particular specificity that can leave a person feeling unsure of exactly what to do. Fortunately, several practices can create a clear plan of how to achieve mental toughness. These practices are like the actual recipes and exercises needed to eat right and get plenty of exercise. By applying these practices, you will begin to develop mental toughness in everything you do, and in every environment, you find yourself in.

Keep Your Emotions in Check

The quest for developing mental toughness is to keep your emotions in check. People who fail to take control of their feelings allow their emotions to control them. More often than not, this takes the form of people who are driven by rage, fear, or both. Whenever people allow their emotions to control them, they let their emotions control their decisions, words, and actions. However, when you keep your emotions in check, you control your choices, terms, and activities, thereby taking control of your life overall.

To keep your emotions in check, you have to learn to subside your emotions before reacting to a situation. Therefore, instead of speaking when you are angry, or making a decision when you are frustrated, take a few minutes to allow your emotions to settle down. Take a moment to sit down, breathe deeply, and let your energies to restore balance. Only when you feel calm and in control should you decide, speak your mind, or take any action.

Practice Detachment

Another critical element for mental toughness is what is known as detachment. This is when you remove yourself emotionally from the particular situation that is going on around you. Even if the condition affects you directly, remaining detached is a very positive thing. The most significant benefit of detachment is that it prevents an emotional response to the job at hand. This is particularly helpful when things are not going according to plan.

Practicing detachment requires a great deal of effort at first. After all, most people are programmed to feel emotionally attached to the events going on around them at any given time. One of the best ways to practice detachment is to tell yourself that the situation isn't permanent. What causes a person to feel fear and frustration when faced with a negative situation is that they think the job is permanent. When you realize that even the worst events are temporary, you avoid the negative emotional response they can create.

Another way to become detached is to determine why you feel attached to the situation in the first place. As long as you don't feed into their negativity, you won't experience the pain they are trying to cause. This is true for anything you encounter. By not feeding a negative situation or event with negative emotions, you prevent that situation from connecting to you. This allows you to exist within a negative game without being affected by it.

Accept What Is Beyond Your Control

Acceptance is one of the cornerstones of mental toughness. This can take the form of accepting yourself for who you are and accepting others for who they are, but it can also take the way of receiving what is beyond your control. When you learn to accept the things you can't change, you rewrite how your mind reacts to every situation you encounter. The matter is that the majority of stress and anxiety felt by the average person results from not being able to change certain things. Once you learn to accept those things you can't change, you eliminate all of that harmful stress and anxiety permanently.

While accepting what is beyond your control will take a little practice, it is quite easy. The trick is to ask yourself if you can do anything at all to change the situation at hand. If the answer is "no," let it go. Rather than wasting time and energy fretting about what you can't control, adopt the mantra, "It is what it is." This might seem careless at first, but after a while, you will realize that it is a real sign of mental strength. By accepting what is beyond your control, you conserve your energy, thoughts, and time for

184

those things you can affect, thereby making your efforts more effective and worthwhile.

Always Be Prepared

Another way to build mental toughness is always to be ready. If you allow life to take you from one event to another, you will feel lost, uncertain, and unprepared for the experiences you encounter. However, when you take the time to prepare yourself for what lies ahead, you will develop a feeling of control over the situation. There are two ways to be ready, and they are equally crucial for developing mental toughness.

The first way to be prepared is to prepare your mind at the beginning of every day. This takes the form of you taking time in the morning to focus your mind on who you are, and your outlook on life in general. Whether you refer to this time as mediation, contemplation, or daily affirmations, the basic principle is the same. You focus your mind on what you believe in and the qualities you aspire to. This will keep you grounded in your ideals throughout the day, helping you to make the right choices regardless of what life throws your way.

The second way to always be prepared is to take the time to prepare yourself for the situation at hand. Give yourself plenty of time to prepare for it. If you have to give a presentation, go over the information you want to present, choose the materials you want to use, and even take the time to make sure you have the exact clothes you want. When you go into a situation fully prepared, you increase your self-confidence, giving you an added edge. Additionally, you will eliminate the stress and anxiety that results from feeling unprepared.

Take the Time to Embrace Success

One of the problems many negatively-minded people experience is that they never take the time to appreciate progress when it comes their way. Sometimes they are too afraid of jinxing that success actually to recognize it. However, most of the time, they are unable to embrace success because their mindset is too negative for such affirmative action. By contrast, mentally healthy people always take the time to embrace the successes that come their way. This serves to build their sense of confidence as well as their feeling of satisfaction with how things are going.

Next time you experience success of any kind, make sure you take a moment to recognize it. You can create an obvious statement, such as going out for drinks, treating yourself to a nice lunch, or some similar expression of gratitude. Alternatively, you can take a quiet moment to reflect on the success and all the effort that went into making it happen. There is no right or wrong way to embrace prosperity, you need to find a way that works for you. The trick to embracing success is not letting it go to your head. Rather than praising your efforts or actions, appreciate the fact that things went well. Also, be sure to appreciate those whose help contributed to your success.

Be Happy with **What You Have**

Contentment is another element that is critical for mental toughness. To develop happiness, you have to learn how to be satisfied with what you have. This doesn't mean that you eliminate ambition or the desire to achieve greater success. Instead, you show gratitude for the positives that currently exist. After all, the only way you will be able to appreciate the fulfillment of your dreams truly is if you can first understand your life the way it is.

One example of this is learning to appreciate your job. This is true whether you like your job or not. Even if you hate your job and desperately want to find another one, always take the time to appreciate the fact that you have a job in the first place. You could be jobless, which would create all sorts of problems in your life. So, even if you hate your job, learn to appreciate it for what it is. This goes for everything in your life. No matter how good or bad a thing is, always enjoy having it before striving to change.

Be Happy with **Who You Are**

In addition to appreciating what you have, you should always be satisfied with who you are. Again, this doesn't mean that you should settle for who you are and not try to improve your life. Instead, it means that you should learn to appreciate who you are. There will always be issues that you want to fix in your life, and things you know you could do better. The problem is that if you focus on the wrong things, you will always see yourself in a negative light. However, when you learn to appreciate the right parts of your personality, you can pursue self-improvement with a sense of pride, hope, and optimism for who you will become as you begin to fulfill your true potential.

Chapter 27: Relaxation Techniques

Since we have seen that emotions are the first obstacle to a healthy and correct relationship with food, we are going to look specifically at the most suitable techniques to appease them. Not only that, these techniques are very important to make hypnosis deeply effective to achieve the desired goals.

In fact, autogenic training is one of the techniques of self-hypnosis. What does self-hypnosis mean? As the word suggests, it is a form of self-induced hypnosis. Beyond the various techniques available, all have the objective of concentrating a single thought object. To say it seems easy, but it is incredible how, in reality, our mind is constantly distracted and even overlaps distant thoughts between them. This leads to emotional tension with repercussions in everyday life.

Other self-hypnosis techniques that we will not deal with in-depth include Benson's and Erickson's.

Benson's is inspired by oriental transcendental meditation. It is based on the constant repetition of a concept to favor a great concentration. Specifically, he recommends repeating the word that evokes the concept several times. It is the easiest and fastest technique ever. It really takes 10-15 minutes a day. Just because it's so simple doesn't mean it's not effective. And you will also need to familiarize yourself with it. Especially for those who are beginners with self-hypnosis. In fact, this could be the first technique to try right away to approach this type of practice.

You sit with your eyes closed in a quiet room and focus on breathing and relax the muscles. Therefore continually think about the object of meditation. If your thought turns away, bring it back to the object. To be sure to practice this self-hypnosis for at least 10 minutes, just set a timer.

Erickson's is apparently more complex. The first step involves creating a new self-image that you would like to achieve. So we start from something we don't like about ourselves and mentally create the positive image that we would like to create.

In our specific case, we could start from the idea of us being overweight and transform that idea into an image of us in perfect shape, satisfied with ourselves in front of the mirror.

Then we focus on three objects around the subject, then three noises, and finally three sensations. It takes little time to concentrate on these things. Gradually decrease this number. Therefore two objects, two noises, and two sensations. Better if the objects are small and with light and unusual sensations, to which little attention is paid. For example, the feeling of the shirt that we wear in contact with our skin. You get to one, and then you leave your mind wandering. We take the negative image we have and calmly transform it mentally into the positive one. At the end of this practice, you will feel great energy and motivation.

Autogenic Training

Autogenic training is a highly effective self-induced relaxation technique without external help. It is called "training" because it includes a series of exercises that allow the gradual and passive acquisition of changes in muscle tone, vascular function, cardiac and pulmonary activity, neuro-vegetative balance, and state of consciousness. But don't be frightened by this word. His exercises do not require a particular theoretical preparation nor a radical modification of one's habits. Practicing this activity allows you to live a profound and repeatable experience at all times.

Autogenic means "self-generating," unlike hypnosis and self-hypnosis, which are actively induced by an operator or the person himself.

In essence, the goal is to achieve inner harmony so that we can best face the difficulties of everyday life. It is a complementary tool for hypnosis. The two activities are intertwined. Practicing both of them allows a better overall experience. In fact, hypnosis helps well to act directly on the subconscious. But for hypnosis to be effective, it is necessary to have already prepared an inner calm such that there is no resistance to the instructions given by the hypnotherapist. The origins of autogenic training are rooted in the activity of hypnosis. In the latter, there is an exclusive relationship between hypnotist and hypnotized. Those who are hypnotized must, therefore, be in a state of maximum receptivity to be able to reach a state of constructive passivity in order to create the ideal relationship with the hypnotist.

Those who approach autogenic training and have already undergone hypnosis sessions can deduce the main training guidelines from the principles of hypnosis. The difference is that you become your own hypnotist. You must, therefore, assume an attitude of receptive availability towards you. Such activity also allows a higher spiritual introspection, feeling masters of one's emotional state. This undoubtedly brings countless advantages in everyday life.

So I usually suggest everyone try a hypnosis session and then do a few days of autogenic training before they start using hypnosis again daily. It's the easiest way to approach the relaxation techniques on your own and start to become familiar with the psycho-physical sensations given by these practices. Mine is a spontaneous suggestion. If you have tried meditation and relaxation techniques in the past you can also go directly into guided hypnosis. In any case, autogenic training can be useful regardless of the level of familiarity with these practices. It is clear that if you have little time in your days, it makes no sense to put so much meat on the fire. Let's remember that they are still relaxation techniques. If we see them too much as "training," we could associate obligations and bad emotions that go against the principle of maximum relaxation. So I'm not saying do autogenic training and hypnosis every day, 10 push-ups, crunches, and maybe yoga, and then you will be relaxed and at peace with your body. This approach is not good. It is about finding your balance and harmony in a practice that has to be pleasant and deliberate.

Basic Autogenic Training Exercises

The basic exercises of the A.T. are classically divided into six exercises of which two are fundamental and four are complementary. Before the six exercises, you practice an induction to calm and relaxation, while at the end recovery and then awakening.

These exercises are considered as consecutive phases to be carried out in each session. It is not mandatory to carry out all the steps together. Especially initially, each exercise will have to be understood individually. But if you intend to stop, for example, in the fourth exercise, and not do all of them, you will necessarily have to do the other 3 exercises in the same session first. The duration of the session remains unchanged, however, because when you add exercises, you will make each phase last less.

First Exercise—"The Heaviness." It s a very useful exercise to overcome psychophysical problems related to muscular tensions that derive from emotional tensions.

Second Exercise—"The heat." It serves to relieve circulatory problems, in all cases where there is a problem of reduced blood flow to the extremities.

Third Exercise—"The Heart." It is a highly suggestive exercise that allows you to regain contact with that part of the body that we traditionally deal with emotions.

Fourth Exercise—"The Breath." It produces better oxygenation of the blood and organs.

Fifth Exercise—"The Solar Plexus." It helps a lot of those who suffer from digestive problems.

Sixth Exercise—"The Fresh Forehead." Produces a brain constriction vessel that can be very useful to reduce headaches, especially if linked to physical or mental overload.

Recommended Positions

The following positions are suitable for both autogenic training and hypnosis and relaxation techniques in general. I suggest initially to use the lying down position and to use it later in hypnosis for virtual gastric bandaging to simulate the position on the surgical couch.

Lie Down

This position, at least at the beginning, is the most used for its comfort. You lie on your back (face up) and your legs slightly apart with your toes out. The arms are slightly detached from the torso and are slightly bent. The fingers are detached from each other and slightly arched.

On the Armchair

You sit with a chair attached to the wall. Your back is firmly against the backrest, and your head rests against the wall. You can place a cushion between your head and the wall.

Alternatively, you can use a high chair to rest your head-on. The feet should be flat firmly on the floor, with a 90-degree angle on the legs. The tips of the feet should be placed on the outside. The arms should be resting on the supports (where present) or the thighs.

If there are supports, the hands should be left dangling.

If they are not present, the hands are resting on the legs, and the fingers are separate.

Position of the Coachman
This position allows you to be seated but without particular basic support. It can be practiced wherever you have something to sit on (a chair, a stone, a stool...).

You sit, for example, on the chair very far forward without leaning forward with your back.

Your feet must be flat firmly on the ground, with the tips pointing outwards. Your back should bend forward by resting your forearms on your thighs and letting your hands dangle between your legs so that they do not touch each other. Pivot your neck forward as much as possible, and relax your shoulders and jaw.

Other Suggestions
To achieve the best results, the environment must be quiet, the phone and any form of technological distraction must be disconnected beforehand. In the room, there must be a very soft light with a constant temperature that allows neither hot nor cold. The environmental conditions, in fact, influence our mood, and the acquisition of a correct position guarantees an objective relaxation of all the muscles.

Do not wear clothes that tighten and restrict your movement: for this purpose also remove the watch and glasses and loosen the belt.

Constancy is very important for achieving a psychic balance. It only takes 10 minutes a day, but a real reluctance is to be taken into consideration. Before doing this practice, you really need to give yourself some time. It must be a deliberate practice. This is one of the reasons why it is not advisable to practice it in small time gaps between commitments, but rather in dedicated time slots.

Also, it is advisable not to practice the exercises immediately after lunch to avoid sleep. At the end of each workout, perform awakening exercises except for the evening just before going to sleep.

At first, checking the relaxation of the various parts of the body will require some reflection. But over time and practice, everything will become more instinctive. Do not expect great results in the first days of practice. Do not abandon the practice the right way because like anything else you cannot expect to know how to do it immediately.

One last tip is to not be too picky when it comes to checking the position to take. In fact, the indications provided are broad; it is not necessary to interpret them rigidly.

Conclusion

This process requires willpower, strength, and discipline. Ensure that you are able to incorporate these into your life to see the results you've only been fantasizing about in the past. Pair this with other meditation books as well to get a variety of brain training that will keep you focused on your biggest dreams.

Your attitude can be one of those major things keeping you from reaching your fitness goals. Being on a healthy kick is not necessary for sustainable weight loss.

Losing weight is surely an amazing goal, but it is extremely hard to reach if there is no good motivation to encourage you to keep going.

It absolutely takes some time to reach that ideal weight, both time and effort, and to motivate yourself on this journey, the best idea is to embrace positive self-talk.

You need to remind yourself of all of the amazing health benefits of losing weight such as feeling more energized, feeling better about yourself, having better sleep, and much more.

In addition to reminding yourself of all of the amazing health benefits of losing weight, another great idea is to keep a success journal where you will write every single step you have taken and succeeded in.

This way, you're more likely to stay committed to your weight loss journey. In order to boost your commitment, you also need to embrace some positive affirmations and positive self-talk which will keep you going.

Therefore, the next time you look yourself in the mirror, instead of telling yourself "I will never be thin and I will just give up," say to yourself "this is going to be amazing, losing those five pounds feels great and I will keep going."

Both of these statements are self-talk, but the first one is extremely negative self-talk while the second one is positive self-talk.

These are automatic statements or thoughts to make to yourself consciously. Positive self-talk is an extremely important step as it can influence how you act or how you feel.

Instead of saying to yourself negative statements, embrace positive affirmations that come with some constructive idea.

Once there, your positive self-talk can act as your own personal guardian angel destroying that annoying, destructive devil that has been sitting on your shoulder keeping you from reaching your goals.

If you have battled to stay on the right track in the past, this is mostly due to that annoying negative self-talk which, once there, brings failure, so you are more likely just to give up.

For this reason, say yes to positive self-talk. The most powerful thing about embracing positive self-talk is that those positive affirmations and positive statements you say to yourself tend to stick in your mind, so you are surrounded by positive feelings and thoughts.

In order to start practicing positive self-talk, you need to start listening to what is happening in your mind and recognize your feelings, desires, and fears as these influence your weight loss journey.

The best idea is to keep a weight loss journal where you will write down what you eat that day, how many hours you exercised as well as your feelings and thoughts throughout the day.

If some negative statements are circling in your head, make sure you write them down. Once you have written them, you need to turn them into affirmations or positive self-talk where instead of "I can't" or "I won't," you say "I can" and "I will."

As you embrace positive self-talk, you are more likely to stay on the right track. Moreover, as you reshape your negative self-talk into positive self-talk, you also get to change your unique self-definition from a person who cannot achieve something to a person who can achieve anything.